# Ul... Smoothies

*Delicious Recipes for*
*Over 125 of the*
*Best Smoothies,*
*Freezes, and Blasts*

Donna Pliner Rodnitzky

**PRIMA PUBLISHING**

Published by Prima Publishing, Roseville, California. Member of the Crown Publishing Group, a division of Random House, Inc.

PRIMA PUBLISHING and colophon are trademarks of Random House, Inc., registered with the United States Patent and Trademark Office.

A per serving nutritional breakdown is provided for each recipe. If a range is given for an ingredient amount, the breakdown is based on the smaller number. If a range is given for servings, the breakdown is based on the larger number. If a choice of ingredients is given in an ingredient listing, the breakdown is calculated using the first choice. Nutritional content may vary depending on the specific brands or types of ingredients used. "Optional" ingredients or those for which no specific amount is stated are not included in the breakdown. Nutritional figures are rounded to the nearest whole number.

**Warning—disclaimer**
This book is not intended to provide medical advice and is sold with the understanding that the publisher and the author are not liable for the misconception or misuse of information provided. The author and Random House, Inc., shall have neither liability nor responsibility to any person or entity with respect to any loss, damage, or injury caused or alleged to be caused directly or indirectly by the information contained in this book or the use of any products mentioned.

*Interior illustrations by Sheryl Dickert*

**Library of Congress Cataloging-in-Publication Data**

Rodnitzky, Donna.
  Ultimate smoothies: delicious recipes for over 125
  of the best smoothies, freezes, and blasts / Donna
  Pliner Rodnitzky.
    p.   cm.
  Includes index.
  ISBN 0-7615-2575-0
  1. Blenders (Cookery).  2. Smoothies (Beverages).
  I. Title.
  TX840.B5 R63   2000
  641.8'75—dc21                                   00-037355
                                                        CIP

02  03  04  05  HH  10  9  8  7  6
Printed in the United States of America
First Edition

**Visit us online at www.primapublishing.com**

*To my husband, Bob, whom I owe my greatest thanks and appreciation for always being there when I need him most, and for never faltering in his confidence in me. And to my children, David, Adam, and Laura, who continue to astound me with their quest for knowledge and their desire to be the best in all they do.*

# Contents

# Preface

Like the yogurt craze of the 1980s, smoothies became one of the success stories of the 1990s and into the new millennium. This is not to say that smoothies are a new phenomenon. When the home blender was introduced in the 1940s, people soon learned that they could combine fruit and ice in it to make a great fruit concoction. As early as the 1960s, health food stores on the West Coast were selling smoothies. More recently, the widespread popularity of these refreshing creations has become increasingly obvious with the proliferation of smoothie shops everywhere across the nation. You will also find smoothies highlighted on menus of eating establishments ranging from yogurt or ice cream shops, to juice bars, to trendy restaurants. Take a stroll down the ice cream aisle of your local supermarket, and you will find commercially made smoothies. But the smoothie revolution isn't confined to shops and restaurants. The sheer number of blender models available speaks volumes of smoothie enthusiasts' desire to create these flavorful drinks in the comfort of their own homes.

Smoothies not only are delicious and healthful taste treats in a glass, but making them also provides an opportunity to showcase your creative talents. With this book as a guide, you will discover how easy it is to transform a fabulous combination of fruits, fruit juices, and dairy products into a mouthwatering temptation. I hope that after a while you will attempt to experiment by substituting or eliminating an ingredient in a recipe and experience the delight of creating your own signature smoothies. For example, if you're lactose intolerant, use a lactose-free product instead of milk, or if you have sugar sensitivity, use unsweetened fruit juices.

*Ultimate Smoothies* was written for all smoothie lovers who savor the delicious and exotic flavors of fresh fruits, as well as the health benefits derived from them. Whether you are a new recruit to the smoothie army or a certified smoothie maven, you will be delighted with all the temptingly delicious recipes found in this book and surprised at how easy and exciting they are to prepare. Along with the recipes you'll find helpful general information, including a description of the wide variety of blenders available to help you choose the one that will meet your needs, a discussion of the fruits that are best for preparing a smoothie, and information on how to increase a smoothie's health benefits. Finally, helpful preparation hints are provided so that each smoothie will be a glass of perfection.

In creating this cookbook, I aimed to provide a contemporary collection of flavorful recipes that would be exciting, fun to read, and easy to prepare. If you crave excitement, don't overlook your blender. Just flip the switch and whir your way to a flavorful, refreshing ecstasy.

# Acknowledgments

I would like to thank Susan Silva, my acquisitions editor, for her encouragement to write *Ultimate Smoothies* and her confidence in my ability to create a book that would meet the high standards of Prima Publishing. I would also like to thank my project editor, Michelle McCormack, for her attention to detail and her excellent suggestions. Thanks to Monica Thomas, cover designer; Sheryl Dickert, illustrator; and the entire staff at Prima Publishing for their outstanding professionalism in bringing this book to publication.

# Introduction

Smoothies are the "in" drink. Whether you drink them for the sheer pleasure of indulging in a refreshing taste sensation or enjoy them as meals in a glass, smoothies have become the ultimate way to quickly satisfy a craving for something delicious and filling.

One of the core reasons for the smoothie craze is that these refreshing creations are composed of the simplest ingredients. The most basic smoothie is made with a combination of fruit, fruit juice, and ice. Beyond the basics, a dairy product, such as milk or yogurt, can be substituted for the juice or included as an additional ingredient. And with such a wide variety of seasonal fruits and juices available year-round, smoothies can be blended into an infinite number of delectable combinations.

People adore smoothies not only because these drinks are inherently delicious but also because they provide certain health benefits. Depending on their ingredients, smoothies are chock-full of vitamins from the fruit, and calcium from the dairy ingredients. Many smoothies are low in fat and calories but still capable of easily appeasing a food craving. Another kudo for smoothies is that these delightful drinks can be supplemented with a wide variety of healthful additives that quickly transform them into an even more nutritionally balanced and wholesome meal.

*Ultimate Smoothies* is a collection of over 125 entertaining recipes that were created to excite your taste buds and put a smile on your face. In this book, I hope to convince you that preparing smoothies is a fun and exciting experience. *Ultimate Smoothies* begins by providing you with all the information necessary to make your smoothie experience successful. In the first few chapters, you will learn what essential equipment is needed to make your kitchen qualify as smoothie central, as well as detailed information on how to select, prepare, and store the best fruits for making a smoothie. Finally, you will be delighted with the host of helpful techniques provided that will enable every smoothie you prepare to become a signature masterpiece.

Chapter 4, "Back to Basics: Classic Smoothie Favorites," will appeal to all smoothie lovers. These smoothies are quick and easy to prepare but are exceptionally tasty because of their richly flavored fruit and fruit juice ingredients. All you need to do to make a basic smoothie is add a complement of your favorite fruit juice, fruit, and ice to a blender and rev it up. For starters, try Blueberry Chill made with a blend of blueberries, bananas, and apple cider. For a real winner, spin the wheel and solve the puzzle of Vanna Banana, made with orange juice, bananas, and strawberries.

Chapter 5, "S*mooooo*thies! Dairy Can Be Merry," will introduce you to a host of delectable smoothies that are made with dairy products, such as milk and yogurt. Dairy ingredients give smoothies a creamier consistency and richer flavor. In most of the recipes, I suggest using lowfat or fat-free dairy products to keep the fat content to a minimum. However, depending on your diet, whole dairy products with fat can be substituted, or ones that are fat-free can be replaced with lowfat ingredients, and vice versa. Any of these substitutions will not appreciably change the taste or consistency of the smoothie. So treat yourself to a glass of Caramel Apple on a Stick, which is a luscious blend of apples, apple juice, vanilla fat-free frozen yogurt, and caramel topping—this is a real old-fashioned treat.

Chapter 6, "R$_X$ Smoothies: Drink to Your Health," contains many recipes made with soy products, as well as several others that feature the addition of health supplements. Although smoothies usually provide a healthy dose of vitamins and calcium derived from their fruit and dairy ingredients, they do not necessarily qualify as a nutritionally complete meal replacement. You will find how easy it is to remedy this by adding health-enhancing powders and supplements, all without substantially changing the drink's taste or texture. For example, you will learn that to enhance protein and iron content, many of the recipes made with ingredients such as lowfat milk or yogurt can be readily substituted with your favorite soy ingredient. You might notice a slight change in the taste, especially if you don't use these ingredients regularly, but the end result will be a tantalizing nutritious smoothie that you can enjoy any time of the day. If you are looking for a boost of energy, try a refreshing glass of Bee

Healthy Raspberry Smoothie. It is a delectable mixture of soy milk, raspberries, bananas, vanilla fat-free frozen yogurt, and bee pollen—a combination that will definitely have you buzzing.

If you want an excuse to break your diet, look no further than chapter 7 entitled "Outrageously Decadent: Indulgence in a Glass." Smoothies can be made with a host of rich ingredients, such as ice cream, chocolate fudge sauce, and many other sinful additions that we usually do not associate with these drinks. Although these smoothies are meant to be an occasional indulgence, keep in mind that you can substitute fat-free or lowfat yogurts for ice cream, and many other suggested lowfat substitutes can be considered as well. If you like halvah, you will be dancing over the recipe for Halvah-Nagila Smoothie. It is a luscious combination of halvah, milk, banana, and cashew crunch ice cream.

Chapter 8, "Black Tie Only: Smoothies Go Uptown," includes recipes for smoothies that were designed to be served on those occasions when a special treat is in order. Dressed up with alcohol and a suggested garnish, these smoothies can grace an elegant dessert plate or be enjoyed on the patio after a candlelight dinner. Although ideal fare to be served up by the butler, these creations are so delicious that I hope you will not limit them only to special occasions. If you are looking for a unique smoothie that is certain to impress your friends, offer them a cocktail glass filled with a Won't You Come Home Banana Bailey smoothie, a creamy blend of banana, Baileys Original Irish

Cream, milk, and vanilla frozen yogurt. Don't forget to garnish it with a Pirouette cookie or Espresso Brittle Shard, which you'll find with the other delicious garnishes in chapter 9, "Garnishes with a Flourish."

Whether you prefer your smoothies with fruit and fruit juices alone or like to add dairy ingredients, fudge sauce, or wheat germ, this book is certain to please you. If you can slice a banana and press the "on" button of your blender, you can become a smoothiemeister.

# Health Benefits of Smoothies

Smoothies are definitely the "in" food for the new millennium, not only because they taste good but because they're good for you. They are exceedingly high in flavor and low in calories and fat, and they can be readily combined with a wide variety of healthful additives. If a more healthful diet is what you're seeking, you need look no further than the ultimate smoothie. Over the years, the National Cancer Institute has actively campaigned to encourage people to include two to three servings of fruit in their diets each day to reduce the risks of a wide variety of serious ailments, such as cancer, arthritis, and heart disease. As scientists have learned more about the bounty of antioxidants found in fresh fruits, it has become increasingly apparent how important it is to enrich our diets with these nutrient-packed powerhouses. By eating fruit, we also benefit from its rich source of carbohydrates, fiber, and minerals.

Although it is not recommended that you consume a smoothie as a complete meal replacement, it can readily become one when protein supplements are added. With the addition of one or more health-enhancing supplements, such as herbs and extracts, a smoothie can quickly become an even more healthful beverage.

Are you craving more energy, hoping to improve your memory, or interested in warding off a cold, or do you simply want to include more health-enhancing soybean products in your diet? Here are some examples of the many wellness-promoting smoothie boosters that can help you achieve these goals:

- **Bee Pollen**
  This natural substance is thought to increase sexual performance and stamina. This protein-rich additive contains twenty-seven minerals, most of the known vitamins, and many enzymes.

- **Brewers Yeast**
  This single-cell organism is an excellent source of vegetarian protein and rich in major B vitamins. It also contains nineteen amino acids and iron.

- **Echinacea**
  An herb that boosts the immune system; it's especially helpful when you are ailing from a cold.

- **Flaxseed Oil**
  Flaxseed oil is an excellent vegetarian source of omega-3 fatty acids and provides essential fatty acids required for a balanced diet.

- **Gingko Biloba**
  This extract comes from the fan-shaped leaf of the gingko tree. It is thought to increase blood flow to the brain, thereby enhancing several of its functions, such as memory.

- **Ginseng**
  Another herb believed to be capable of normalizing various bodily functions, increasing mental alertness and vitality, relieving stress, and enhancing immunity.

- **Lecithin**
  Lecithin is a nutrient compound derived from soybean oil. It is believed to play a role in maintaining cardiovascular health and aiding liver and cell function.

- **Oat Bran**
  Oat bran contains B vitamins, minerals, and proteins. It is an excellent source of fiber.

- **Protein Powders**
  Most often soy based, protein powders provide a natural source of amino acids, vitamins, minerals, fiber, and iron.

- **Soy Milk and Soy Yogurt**
  Soy milk is made from soybeans that are soaked, finely ground, and strained, while soy yogurt is made from soy milk. These foods are an excellent source of high quality protein, B vitamins, and iron. In addition, a diet

that is low in saturated fats and rich with soy foods is believed to lower LDL ("bad") cholesterol levels.

- **Wheat Germ**
  Wheat germ is rich in insoluble fiber as well as six essential vitamins and minerals, including vitamin E.

So, the next time you are looking for some quick and easy refreshment that is also packed with power boosters, look no further than your own kitchen countertop. Simply by adding any of the suggested herbs, plant derivatives, or protein powders to smoothie ingredients in your blender, you can have an energy-packed glassful that is as nutritious as it is delicious. To your health!

# CHAPTER 2

# The Incomparable Fruit

## How to Select, Prepare, and Store Fresh Fruit

When it comes to making smoothies, being well-informed about the wide variety of fruits available for creating the perfect smoothie is as important as purchasing the right blender (which we'll discuss in the next chapter). You will be pleasantly surprised to discover how easy it is to determine whether these delectable packages of flavor are ripe or not. Which fruits should be gently pressed to determine their resilience or softness? Why does the weight or density of specific fruits indicate their degree of juiciness or ripeness? How does simply smelling a fruit and basking in its sweet aroma help determine its ripeness? Read on to unravel these and other mysteries of the produce department.

I hope that as you become more familiar with the fabulous array of fruit available, the excitement of making smoothies will inspire you to create your own recipes with some of your favorite fruit that I may not have included. With such a delicious bounty of fruit to choose from, this is going to be one of the tastiest adventures of your life.

# APPLES

Apples are believed to have originated in Central Asia and Caucasus, but they have been cultivated since prehistoric times. They were brought to the United States at the beginning of the seventeenth century and later to Africa and Australia. Today, there are over 100 varieties of apples commercially grown in the United States.

Apples are a small, round fruit that can be red, green, or yellow. They have a firm, crisp flesh. Some apples have a sweet flavor with a hint of tartness, while others are less sweet and more tart. Most apples are delicious when made into a smoothie, but your flavor preference will determine the best one for you.

## Selection

When choosing an apple, look for one that is firm and crisp with a smooth and tight skin. Most important, the apple should have a sweet-smelling aroma. Avoid any apple that has bruised or blemished skin. Another consideration when choosing apples is to buy the organic variety whenever possible. Most nonorganic apples are heavily sprayed with pesticides and later waxed to preserve and keep them looking fresh. Because of this, you might find a worm in some organic apples. These unwelcome visitors can be removed when the apple is cut, thereby removing any health or aesthetic concerns. Wash and dry all apples well, whether organic or not.

## APRICOTS

The apricot is a round or oblong fruit measuring about two inches in diameter with skin and flesh that are orange-yellow in color. It is a very sweet and juicy fruit with a single, smooth stone. The apricot is native to North China and was known to be a food source as early as 2200 B.C. Apricots are an excellent source of vitamin A, potassium, and iron.

### Selection

When choosing apricots, look for those that are well-colored and firm but yield slightly when gently pressed. Avoid any that are green or yellow in color because this may indicate they are not ripe, while soft ones are probably overripe. Wash apricots and keep them refrigerated until ready to use.

## BANANAS

The banana has been around for so long that, according to Hindu legend, it was actually the forbidden fruit of the Garden of Eden. It is also believed that the banana was widely cultivated throughout Asia and Oceania before recorded history and that the Spanish colonists introduced banana shoots to the New World in 1516. Bananas are a rich source of vitamins A, B, C, and $B_2$, as well as potassium.

## Selection

Although bananas are picked when they are green, they are not allowed to ripen until they get to market. When choosing a banana, look for one that is completely yellow. The riper a banana, or the more yellow its skin, the sweeter it is. Bananas that are yellow but have green tips or are yellow with brown spots also are ready to eat. Green bananas will ripen at room temperature in two or three days, or you can place them in a brown paper bag to ripen. If you add a tomato or apple to the bag, the bananas will ripen even faster. Once ripe, store bananas at room temperature or in the refrigerator for a couple of days.

# BLACKBERRIES

The blackberry is a small black, blue, or dark red berry that grows on thorny bushes (brambles). These berries are oblong in shape and grow up to one inch in length. The United States is the world's dominant producer of blackberries. Blackberries are at their peak in flavor and availability from June through September, but they may still be found in some supermarkets from November and on into April. They are rich in vitamin C and fiber.

## Selection

When choosing blackberries, look for ones that are plump and solid with full color and a bright, fresh appearance.

# BLUEBERRIES

Native to North America, the blueberry has the distinction of being the second most popular berry in the United States. It has been around for thousands of years but was not cultivated until the turn of the century. Today, 95 percent of the world's commercial crop of blueberries is grown in the United States. Blueberries are at their peak in flavor from mid-April to late September. They are available in the southern states first and gradually move north as the season progresses. Blueberries are an excellent source of vitamin C and fiber.

## Selection

When choosing blueberries, look for ones that are plump and firm. Avoid any that appear to be dull because this may indicate that the fruit is old.

# CHERRIES

Cherries are small, round, red to black fruit that grow on a tree. There are numerous varieties, but all of them fall into one of three categories: sweet, sour, or a hybrid of the two. Cherries grow in the temperate zones of Europe, Asia, and the Americas. It is believed that they originated in northeastern Asia and later spread throughout the temperate zones in prehistory carried by birds who ate the cherries and later dropped the stones. They are a source of vitamin C and fiber.

*Selection*

When choosing cherries, look for those that are dark, plump, and firm. Store them in the refrigerator and wash them just before using.

# KIWIFRUIT

The kiwifruit (or kiwi) is about the size of a plum and grows on a vine. It has a brown fuzzy skin and a luscious sweet-and-sour emerald-green pulp that surrounds a cluster of black seeds. The kiwi originated in the 1600s in the Yangtze River valley in China and was called "Yangtao." In 1906, Yangtao seeds were sent to New Zealand, where the fruit was renamed Chinese gooseberry. In 1962, the Chinese gooseberry was shipped to the United States, where it was again renamed the "kiwifruit" in honor of New Zealand's famous national bird. Kiwi is high in vitamin C.

*Selection*

When choosing a kiwi, look for one that has a sweet aroma and is plump and firm, yet will give slightly when pressed. Kiwi will ripen at room temperature in three to five days. When ripe, store the kiwi in the refrigerator for a few days.

# MANGOES

The mango was cultivated in India and the Malay Archipelago about four thousand years ago. In the 1700s and 1800s, European explorers introduced the fruit to other tropical areas.

Mangoes were first grown in the United States sometime in the early 1900s.

The mango resembles a peach in appearance but is more elongated in shape. It has a thin, leathery skin that can be yellow or red in color. The skin surrounds a very aromatic and juicy pulp and a hard inner pit. Mangoes are rich in beta-carotene and vitamins A and C.

## Selection

When choosing a mango, look for one that is very fragrant, plump around the stem area, and gives slightly when pressed. Mangoes can also be ripened at room temperature. Wash and dry them well before using.

# MELONS

Melons, surprisingly, are members of the cucumber family. They grow on vines that can be up to seven feet long. There are two distinct types of melons: muskmelons and watermelons. In the muskmelon category are the summer melons, cantaloupe and muskmelon, and the winter melons, including the casaba and honeydew. All melons are high in vitamin C.

## Selection

When choosing a melon, look for one that is unblemished, firm, and free of any soft spots. Pick up a few melons and choose the one that is the heaviest for its size. Also, smell the stem end of the melon to see whether it has a fresh, melon aroma. If it has no aroma, then the fruit is not ripe. Melons should be washed and refrigerated until ready to use.

# ORANGES

Fresh oranges are widely grown in California, Florida, and Arizona and are available all year long. The two major varieties are the Valencias and navel. Two other varieties grown in the Western states are the Cara Cara navel and the Moro orange (similar to the blood orange), both of which are available throughout the winter months. Oranges are very high in vitamin C.

## Selection

When selecting an orange, look for one that is heavy for its size and firm. Avoid oranges with a bruised skin, indicating possible fermentation, as well as those with a loose skin, suggesting they may be dry inside. Although oranges can be stored at room temperature for a few days, their flavor is best when kept refrigerated. Wash the oranges before storing them.

# PAPAYAS

The papaya has a smooth skin that can be green or greenish yellow in color. It surrounds a flesh that ranges in color from yellow-orange to salmon. It has a slightly elongated shape, similar to that of an avocado, and contains many edible seeds. Its flavor has been described as musky peachy-apricot. Papayas are an excellent source of vitamin C and beta-carotene.

## Selection

When choosing a papaya, look for one that is heavy for its size and gives slightly when pressed. Also, the papaya should have a pleasant aroma. If the skin is spotted, this will not affect the flavor. Papayas are at their peak during May and June. Wash the papaya before using.

# PEACHES AND NECTARINES

Grown since prehistoric times, peaches were first cultivated in China. They were later introduced into Europe and Persia. It is believed that the Spaniards brought peaches to North, Central, and South America. The Spanish missionaries planted the first peach trees in California.

Numerous varieties of peaches are available, and they are broken down into rough classifications. An example of one type of peach is the "freestone," so named because the pit separates easily from the peach. Another type is the "clingstone," because the pit is firmly attached to the fruit. Freestones are most often found in the supermarket because they are easy to eat, while clingstone peaches are frequently canned. Peaches are available almost year-round and are a good source of vitamins A and C.

The nectarine is a smooth-skinned variety of the peach. Nectarines are high in vitamin C.

## Selection

When choosing nectarines, look for those with bright red markings over a yellow skin. Avoid any with wrinkled skin or those that are soft and bruised. The nectarine should yield gently to the touch and have a sweet aroma.

When picking peaches, look for ones that are relatively firm with a fuzzy, creamy yellow skin, and a sweet aroma. The pink blush on the peach indicates its variety, not its ripeness. Avoid peaches with a wrinkled skin or those that are soft or blemished.

The peach should yield gently when touched. To ripen peaches, keep them at room temperature, out of direct sun, until the skin yields slightly to the touch. Once ripe, wash the peaches and store them in the refrigerator in a single layer for up to five days.

# PEARS

Pear is the name of a tree of the rose family and its fruit. It is believed that pears were eaten by Stone Age people. However, the pears we are accustomed to eating were first cultivated in southeastern Europe and western Asia as early as 2000 B.C. Pear trees were first planted in the Americas in the early seventeenth century. Pears are a source of vitamin C and fiber.

## Selection

Although pears are available year-round, they ripen better off the tree. This explains why they are often so hard when purchased at the super-market. Many pears have stickers that tell you the stage of ripeness, such as "ready to eat" or "let me ripen for two days." Therefore, when choosing pears, look for ones that are firm and unblemished with a fresh pear aroma. Pears can then be ripened at home by placing them in a brown paper bag at room temperature for a few days. Once ripe, wash the pears and refrigerate them for two to five days.

# PINEAPPLES

The pineapple is a tropical fruit that is native to Central and South America. In 1493, Christopher Columbus discovered pineapples growing on the island of Guadeloupe and brought them back to Spain. In the 1700s, pineapples were grown in greenhouses throughout Europe. They are an excellent source of vitamin C.

## Selection

When choosing a pineapple, look for one that has a fresh pineapple aroma and a crown with crisp, fresh-looking leaves and a brightly colored shell. Avoid any pineapples that have soft spots or are discolored. Wash the pineapple well.

# RASPBERRIES

It is believed that red raspberries spread all over Europe and Asia in prehistoric times. Because they were so delicious growing wild, it was not until the 1600s that raspberries were cultivated in Europe. Those that are cultivated in North America originated from two groups: the red raspberry, native to Europe, and the wild red variety, native to North America. Raspberries are an excellent source of vitamin C, fiber, and potassium.

## Selection

When choosing raspberries, it is always best to buy them when they are in season—usually starting in late June and lasting four to six weeks. If you are fortunate enough to have a local berry farm, take advantage of it by visiting at the beginning of the season to get the best pick. Select berries that are large and plump, bright, shiny, uniform in color, and free of mold. Avoid any that are mushy. Before refrigerating raspberries for up to one day, carefully go through the batch and discard any that show signs of spoilage. Wash the raspberries just before you are ready to use them.

# STRAWBERRIES

Strawberries date as far back as 2,200 years ago. They are known to have grown wild in Italy in the third century, and by 1588, they were discovered in Virginia by the first European settlers. Local Indians cultivated the strawberry as early as the mid-1600s; by the middle of the nineteenth century, this fruit was widely grown in many parts of the country.

The strawberry grows on a plant very low to the ground on a stem in groups of three. As the fruit ripens, it changes from greenish white in color to a lush flame red. The strawberry does not have a skin but is actually covered by hundreds of tiny seeds. Strawberries are a rich source of vitamin C and fiber.

## Selection

The best time to buy strawberries is in June and July when they are at their peak of juicy freshness.

As with raspberries, if you are lucky enough to live near a strawberry farm, a "pick your own" day trip is a wonderful family outing as well as an excellent way to get the very best of the crop. Look for plump, firm, and deep colored fruit with a bright green cap and a sweet strawberry aroma. Strawberries can be stored in a single layer in the refrigerator for up to two days and washed with their cap just before you are ready to use them.

## FREEZING FRUIT

• Freezing the fruit you plan to include in your smoothie is very important because the frozen fruit adds consistency to the final product and helps maintain an ideal icy cold temperature. Another reason you may want to freeze fruit is simply to store it for later use. Whether freezing for immediate use or for storage, the basic preparation is identical. When ready to freeze cherries and apricots (which should be cut in half and their stones removed) or berries, place them in a colander and rinse with a gentle stream of cool water. Pat dry with a paper towel. For a banana or kiwi, remove its skin and either slice it or freeze it whole and then slice it later before use. Before freezing oranges, remove the peel and as much of the skin as possible, and break each orange into segments. To prepare apples, peaches, nectarines, mangoes, papayas, pears, and melons for freezing, remove their peels and seeds or pits before cubing. When ready to freeze a pineapple, remove its top, the outer layering, and the core, and cut it into cubes.

Place the prepared fruit on a baking sheet, and freeze it for thirty minutes or longer, after which time it will be ready to add to the other smoothie ingredients. If freezing fruit to be used at a later date, transfer the frozen pieces to an airtight plastic bag large enough to hold them in a single layer. Label and mark the date on the bag, and freeze for up to two weeks. Most fruit can be kept in the freezer this long without a loss of flavor. When you are ready to use this deep-frozen fruit, allow it to sit first at room temperature for twenty minutes.

# chapter 3

# Making the Ultimate Smoothie

Equipment and Techniques

You will be delighted to discover just how quick and easy it is to prepare a delicious smoothie. Because many of us are feeling completely overbooked with life's daily responsibilities, spending a lot of time in the kitchen is not always possible. That is why smoothies have become the rage of our era. With very little effort, you can have a satisfying and richly flavored drink within minutes that will put a smile on your face.

A few essential tools are all you need to equip your smoothie operation: a good sharp knife for prepping the fruit, a spatula to remove every last drop of the smoothie from the blender, plastic airtight freezer bags for storing freshly cut fruit in the freezer, and the all-important blender. Although a food processor can be used to make a smoothie, a blender seems to be the preferred appliance for most smoothie mavens.

## EQUIPMENT

The blender is the most important piece of kitchen equipment you will need to make a proper smoothie. The invention of this indispensable appliance is credited to Stephen J. Poplawski who, in 1922, was the first one to place a spinning blade at the bottom of a glass container. By 1935, Fred Waring and Frederick Osius made improvements on the original design and marketed the "Waring Blender." The rest is history.

A blender basically consists of a glass, metal, or plastic food container that is fitted with a metal blade at the bottom. It sits on a base with a control panel that allows the blades to spin at different speeds so that they can liquefy, puree, chop, or whip almost any food that is reasonably soft.

You should assess certain basic qualities when selecting a blender, including its durability, ease of operation and cleaning, and noise production. Once these criteria are met, you are ready to narrow down your choice. With such a wide variety of blenders from which to choose, I hope the information listed here will help in your decision.

• Blender containers typically come in two sizes: thirty-two ounces and forty ounces. If you will routinely be preparing smoothies for more than two people, choose the larger one.

• Blender motors come in different sizes. Those with 290-watt motors are adequate for most blending jobs, but not optimal for smoothies. Others with 330 to 400 watts are considered to be of professional caliber and are excellent for crushing ice, a feature that is very important for creating the best smoothies.

- Blenders can be found with a variety of blade speed options, ranging from two-speed (high and low) to five- and ten-speeds. Variable-speed models provide more options, such as the ability to liquefy and whip.

- The blender should have a removable bottom for ease of cleaning.

- Container lids should have a secondary lid that can be easily removed. This allows for the addition of ingredients while the blender is turned on.

- Avoid plastic container jars because they do not wash well in the dishwasher and therefore must be hand-washed.

Although the blender is most often used to make smoothies, you may prefer the food processor because of its versatility. According to the *New York Times,* the advent of the food processor was the "twentieth-century French revolution." This unique appliance can mince, chop, grate, shred, slice, knead, blend, puree, liquefy, and crush ice.

The food processor has a base directly under the work bowl that houses the motor. A metal shaft extending from the base through the center of the work bowl connects the blade or disc to the motor. A cover that fits over the work bowl has a feed tube. When the bowl is locked into place and the motor is switched on, the shaft turns and propels the blades or discs.

Similar to the blender, the food processor has some basic qualities you should assess when selecting one that best fits your cooking needs.

- Food processors come in a wide range of sizes: the two-cup miniprocessor is practical for chopping, especially small quantities of food; the seven-, nine-, and eleven-cup capacities are each equally suitable for making smoothies, as well as other food preparations; while the fourteen- and twenty-cup units are ideal for professional cooking needs.

- Most food processors have two speeds, high and low, in addition to a pulsing action. (Some food processors have four speeds.)

- Some food processors come with both large and small feed tubes. The larger tube is convenient when large-sized ingredients are to be added while the machine is running.

Once you have decided on the features you would like in a blender or food processor, I highly recommend that you visit several appliance or department stores and personally view the various models available. The salesclerk should be able to provide you with information to further help you in making the best decision. Another resource for gleaning valuable information is the Internet. Many of the companies that manufacture these appliances have sites that are quite informative regarding their individual product, and some also will provide a phone number so you can personally speak to a representative. Finally, *Consumer Reports* and similar publications provide comparison quality ratings of a variety of blenders and food processors.

## HELPFUL TECHNIQUES

Now that the blender is taking center stage on your countertop, it is time to rev it up and make a smoothie. By now you know how easy it is to equip a kitchen with the necessary tools to make smoothies, and you will be delighted to learn that mastering the techniques required to prepare them is just as simple. Preparing a smoothie is probably one of the most uncomplicated tasks you will ever have to perform in your kitchen. I have no doubt that if you were to simply dump all the ingredients in a blender, you could still end up with a perfectly acceptable smoothie. However, for those who want to create the ultimate smoothie, I have included a few helpful techniques that will help you reach this lofty goal.

- To be certain of using the most delicious fruits, buy them when they are in season and at their peak in flavor.

- Before freezing fruit, wash and dry it first, and then follow the preparation instructions given in chapter 2. Placing fruit in the freezer for at least thirty minutes or until partially frozen assures that the smoothie will have both a thick consistency and a rich, fruity flavor.

- Store-bought individually frozen fruit can be substituted for fresh frozen fruit, but it should be used within six months of the purchase date. Avoid using frozen fruit that is packaged in sweetened syrup.

- To keep a supply of your favorite seasonal fruits, stock up before they are no longer available for purchase. Although fruits have the most flavor when kept frozen for only one to two weeks, they can be kept in the freezer for a slightly longer amount of time.

- If using ice in a smoothie, the individual pieces should be slightly smaller than the fruit to prevent any chunks of ice remaining once the smoothie is blended. An easier alternative to cutting the ice is to buy a bag of ice chips or crushed ice to keep in your freezer. If you don't own a high-speed blender, you can make your own crushed ice by simply placing ice cubes in a resealable bag and crushing them with a mallet or rolling pin.

- When adding ingredients to a blender, always add the chilled liquid first, then the frozen fruit, and the ice or frozen yogurt last. Start the blender on low speed to crush the ice and blend the mixture. Gradually increase the speed until the mixture is smooth. It may be necessary to turn the blender off periodically and stir the mixture with a spoon, working from the bottom up.

- If the smoothie is too thin, add more fruit or ice. Conversely, if the smoothie is too thick, add more liquid.

# CHAPTER 4

## Back to Basics

### Classic Smoothie Favorites

*A*merica's love affair with smoothies is easy to understand—they taste good, they're good for you, and they are easy to prepare. Best of all, the ingredient combinations are limitless. In the following pages, you will discover recipes that blend a variety of fruit and juices deliciously. You'll be delighted with Cherry Home Companion, made with apple cider, cherries, and raspberry sorbet; and Watermelon Ecstasy, a combination of pineapple juice, watermelon, and blueberries—to name just a few of these tempting creations.

But keep in mind that the recipes provided here are only a beginning on the road to your ultimate enjoyment of smoothies. Let your imagination take wing by experimenting with other combinations of your favorite fruit and juices, and soon, like an artist splashing colors on a canvas, you will find yourself intermingling interesting tastes and unusual consistencies to create unique world-class smoothies. With one flick of the blender switch, you can become a Picasso of the pineapple!

# A High-Five Freeze

*A smoothie made with five different fruits doesn't get much better.*

### 2 SERVINGS

¼ cup peach nectar (or nectar or juice of your choice)

1 tablespoon honey

¾ cup peeled and diced mango (1 mango)

¾ cup peeled and diced papaya (1 papaya)

¾ cup sliced banana (1 banana)

¾ cup peeled and diced peach (1 peach)

¾ cup diced pineapple (1 pineapple)

½ cup crushed ice

Place the nectar, honey, mango, papaya, banana, peach, pineapple, and ice in a blender, and mix on low speed until the mixture is blended. Continue mixing, gradually increasing the speed, until the mixture is smooth. Pour into glasses and garnish each with a Pineapple Spear (page 208), if desired.

| | | | | |
|---|---|---|---|---|
| Calories | 217 | Calcium | 32 mg |
| Calories from fat | 7 | Iron | 0.70 mg |
| Total fat | 0.02 g | Potassium | 663 mg |
| Carbohydrates | 56 g | Beta Carotene | 1713 mcg |
| Protein | 2 g | Vitamin C | 70 mg |
| Fiber | 6 g | Folic Acid | 48 mcg |

# A Lovely Pear
of Coconuts

*Puns aside, pears and coconut milk make a delightfully exotic smoothie. If you have a spare coconut shell available, serve the smoothie in it and garnish with a wedge of pineapple and a cherry.*

2 SERVINGS

1 cup light coconut milk

1 tablespoon honey

2 cups peeled and diced pear (2 large pears)

1 cup sliced banana (1 large banana)

½ cup lemon sorbet

Place the coconut milk, honey, pear, banana, and sorbet in a blender, and mix on low speed until the mixture is blended. Continue mixing, gradually increasing the speed, until the mixture is smooth. Pour into glasses and garnish each by inserting a Crisp Banana Wafer (page 191) upright in the smoothie, if desired.

| | | | |
|---|---|---|---|
| Calories | 337 | Calcium | 23 mg |
| Calories from fat | 64 | Iron | 1 mg |
| Total fat | 7 g | Potassium | 524 mg |
| Carbohydrates | 73 g | Beta Carotene | 56 mcg |
| Protein | 3 g | Magnesium | 32 mg |
| Fiber | 6 g | Folic Acid | 27 mcg |

# Berry Happy to Meet You

*For friends or family who have never tasted a smoothie, this is the ideal one to make their acquaintance.*

### 2 SERVINGS

¾ cup apple cider

1 tablespoon honey

1½ cups sliced banana (2 large bananas)

1 cup diced strawberries

1 cup blueberries

Place the cider, honey, banana, strawberries, and blueberries in a blender, and mix on low speed until the mixture is blended. Continue mixing, gradually increasing the speed, until the mixture is smooth. Pour into glasses and garnish the rim of each glass with a Strawberry Fan (page 212), if desired.

| | | | | |
|---|---|---|---|---|
| Calories | 241 | Calcium | 29 mg |
| Calories from fat | 11 | Iron | 1 mg |
| Total fat | 1 g | Potassium | 755 mg |
| Carbohydrates | 61 g | Beta Carotene | 111 mcg |
| Protein | 2 g | Magnesium | 47 mg |
| Fiber | 7 g | Vitamin C | 68 mg |

# Blueberry Chill

*You'll find a definite thrill—but not many Fats—when feasting on Blueberry Chill.*

### 2 SERVINGS

1 cup apple cider

1 tablespoon honey

2 cups blueberries

2 cups sliced banana (2 large bananas)

Place the cider, honey, blueberries, and banana in a blender, and mix on low speed until the mixture is blended. Continue mixing, gradually increasing the speed, until the mixture is smooth. Pour into glasses and garnish each with Berries on a Skewer (page 169), if desired.

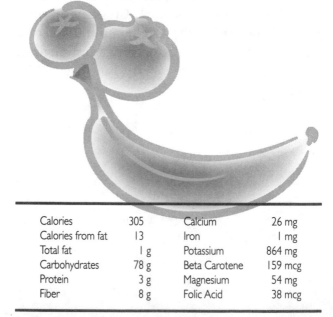

| Calories | 305 | Calcium | 26 mg |
|---|---|---|---|
| Calories from fat | 13 | Iron | 1 mg |
| Total fat | 1 g | Potassium | 864 mg |
| Carbohydrates | 78 g | Beta Carotene | 159 mcg |
| Protein | 3 g | Magnesium | 54 mg |
| Fiber | 8 g | Folic Acid | 38 mcg |

# Cherry Home Companion

*Like all the children in Lake Woebegone, this smoothie is way above average. It is fabulous when cherries are at their ripest. If this delectable fruit is not available fresh and you have a craving for this smoothie, the frozen variety can be substituted.*

## 2 SERVINGS

¾ cup apple cider

1 tablespoon honey

2 cups stemmed and diced Bing cherries

1 cup sliced banana (1 large banana)

¾ cup raspberry sorbet

Place the cider, honey, cherries, banana, and sorbet in a blender, and mix on low speed until the mixture is blended. Continue mixing, gradually increasing the speed, until the mixture is smooth. Pour into glasses and garnish each with fresh mint and a cherry, if desired.

| | | | |
|---|---|---|---|
| Calories | 328 | Calcium | 33 mg |
| Calories from fat | 17 | Iron | 1 mg |
| Total fat | 2 g | Potassium | 774 mg |
| Carbohydrates | 81 g | Beta Carotene | 204 mcg |
| Protein | 3 g | Magnesium | 40 mg |
| Fiber | 5 g | Vitamin C | 23 mg |

# Crazy for You Cranberry Smoothie

*I used my juicer to make a combination of fresh cranberry and grape juice and had about one cup left over, so I devised this recipe. If you don't have fresh juice, just substitute the commercial variety.*

2 SERVINGS

1 cup cranberry-grape juice

1 tablespoon honey

1½ cups raspberries

1½ cup sliced banana (2 large bananas)

½ cup crushed ice

Place the juice, honey, raspberries, banana, and ice in a blender, and mix on low speed until the mixture is blended. Continue mixing, gradually increasing the speed, until the mixture is smooth. Pour into glasses and garnish the rim of each glass with a slice of lime, if desired.

| | | | |
|---|---|---|---|
| Calories | 200 | Calcium | 28 mg |
| Calories from fat | 7 | Iron | 0.64 mg |
| Total fat | 0.82 g | Potassium | 425 mg |
| Carbohydrates | 51 g | Beta Carotene | 64 mcg |
| Protein | 2 g | Magnesium | 37 mg |
| Fiber | 6 g | Vitamin C | 61 mg |

# Go Fly a Papaya

*Get outta here and into the kitchen for some tropical refreshment.*

2 SERVINGS

1 cup orange juice

1½ tablespoons honey

2 cups diced pineapple (1 pineapple)

1 cup peeled and diced papaya (1 large papaya)

1 cup crushed ice

Place the juice, honey, pineapple, papaya, and ice in a blender, and mix on low speed until the mixture is blended. Continue mixing, gradually increasing the speed, until the mixture is smooth. Pour into glasses and garnish each by inserting a Pineapple Chip (page 205) upright in the smoothie, if desired.

| | | | |
|---|---|---|---|
| Calories | 207 | Calcium | 42 mg |
| Calories from fat | 9 | Iron | 0.96 mg |
| Total fat | 1 g | Potassium | 611 mg |
| Carbohydrates | 52 g | Beta Carotene | 99 mcg |
| Protein | 2 g | Vitamin C | 129 mg |
| Fiber | 3 g | Folic Acid | 81 mcg |

# Have Some Com-Passion Fruit

*Be nice . . . be happy . . . live and let live, but don't pass up the opportunity to taste this tropical treat.*

### 2 SERVINGS

1 cup passion fruit nectar

½ tablespoon honey

2 cups diced pineapple (1 pineapple)

2 cups sliced banana (2 large bananas)

1 cup crushed ice

Place the nectar, honey, pineapple, banana, and ice in a blender, and mix on low speed until the mixture is blended. Continue mixing, gradually increasing the speed, until the mixture is smooth. Pour into glasses and garnish the rim of each glass with a Pineapple, Orange, and Cherry Blossom (page 207), if desired.

| | | | |
|---|---|---|---|
| Calories | 313 | Calcium | 23 mg |
| Calories from fat | 13 | Iron | 1 mg |
| Total fat | 1 g | Potassium | 910 mg |
| Carbohydrates | 80 g | Beta Carotene | 90 mcg |
| Protein | 2 g | Magnesium | 74 mg |
| Fiber | 6 g | Vitamin C | 52 mg |

# Kiwi Fusion

*The emerald color of this smoothie speckled with seeds makes it a tempting sight. Once you have tasted it, you'll be glad you were tempted.*

### 2 SERVINGS

¾ cup pineapple juice

½ tablespoon honey

1 cup peeled and diced kiwi (6 kiwi)

1 cup diced pineapple (½ pineapple)

1 cup sliced banana (1 large banana)

Place the juice, honey, kiwi, pineapple, and banana in a blender, and mix on low speed until the mixture is blended. Continue mixing, gradually increasing the speed, until the mixture is smooth. Pour into glasses and garnish the rim of each glass with a slice of kiwi, if desired.

| | | | |
|---|---|---|---|
| Calories | 230 | Calcium | 49 mg |
| Calories from fat | 10 | Iron | 1 mg |
| Total fat | 1 g | Potassium | 806 mg |
| Carbohydrates | 58 g | Beta Carotene | 143 mcg |
| Protein | 2 g | Vitamin C | 116 mg |
| Fiber | 6 g | Folic Acid | 78 mcg |

# Mango in the Morning

*Better than a cup of coffee, this smoothie will jump-start your day.*

### 2 SERVINGS

¾ cup apricot nectar

1 tablespoon honey

1 cup peeled and diced mango or papaya
  (1 large mango or papaya)

1 cup sliced banana (1 large banana)

¾ cup strawberry sorbet

½ cup crushed ice

Place the nectar, honey, mango or papaya, banana, sorbet, and ice in a blender, and mix on low speed until the mixture is blended. Continue mixing, gradually increasing the speed, until the mixture is smooth. Pour into glasses and garnish the rim of each glass with a Strawberry Fan (page 212), if desired.

| | | | |
|---|---|---|---|
| Calories | 308 | Calcium | 25 mg |
| Calories from fat | 8 | Iron | 0.91 mg |
| Total fat | 0.84 g | Potassium | 539 mg |
| Carbohydrates | 79 g | Beta Carotene | 2702 mcg |
| Protein | 2 g | Magnesium | 34 mg |
| Fiber | 0.81 g | Vitamin C | 41 mg |

# Melon Madness

*This refreshingly delicious smoothie can be made with any of your favorite melons. Try it with a combination of two or three.*

### 2 SERVINGS

*8 pitted dates, diced\**

*2 cups passion fruit nectar*

*1 tablespoon honey*

*2 cups seeded and diced mixed melon*

Place the pureed dates with nectar, honey, and melon in a blender and mix on low speed until the mixture is blended. Continue mixing, gradually increasing the speed, until the mixture is smooth. Pour into glasses and garnish each with a Fruit Skewer (page 195), if desired.

**\*To puree dates:** Combine the dates and ½ cup boiling water in a cup; set aside for 15 minutes. Cover the cup with plastic wrap, and refrigerate for several hours or until well chilled. When chilled, drain the dates. Combine the dates and passion fruit nectar in the blender and puree until smooth.

| | | | |
|---|---|---|---|
| Calories | 346 | Calcium | 35 mg |
| Calories from fat | 6 | Iron | 1 mg |
| Total fat | 0.63 g | Potassium | 983 mg |
| Carbohydrates | 90 g | Beta Carotene | 1847 mcg |
| Protein | 3 g | Magnesium | 54 mg |
| Fiber | 4 g | Folic Acid | 56 mcg |

# Orange You Glad You're You

*Drink this smoothie in the morning, and you are certain to start the day with a smile on your face.*

### 2 SERVINGS

1 cup orange juice

½ tablespoon honey

1 cup peeled, seeded and sectioned orange
   (1 large orange)

1 cup peeled and diced mango (1 large mango)

1 cup diced pineapple (½ pineapple)

Place the juice, honey, orange, mango, and pineapple in a blender, and mix on low speed until the mixture is blended. Continue mixing, gradually increasing the speed, until the mixture is smooth. Pour into glasses and garnish the rim of each glass with an Orange Wheel (page 199), if desired.

| | | | |
|---|---|---|---|
| Calories | 206 | Calcium | 64 mg |
| Calories from fat | 8 | Iron | 0.75 mg |
| Total fat | 0.91 g | Potassium | 630 mg |
| Carbohydrates | 52 g | Beta Carotene | 2016 mcg |
| Protein | 2 g | Vitamin C | 145 mg |
| Fiber | 5 g | Folic Acid | 85 mcg |

# Outrageously Orange

*This refreshing glassful is a close cousin of the popular strawberry and banana smoothie. What makes this one special is the addition of oranges and raspberry preserves.*

### 2 SERVINGS

1 cup orange juice

1 tablespoon honey

1 cup peeled, seeded, and sectioned orange
  (1 large orange)

1 cup diced strawberries

1 cup sliced banana (1 large banana)

1 cup crushed ice

2 tablespoons strawberry or raspberry preserves

Place the juice, honey, orange, strawberries, banana, ice, and preserves in a blender, and mix on low speed until the mixture is blended. Continue mixing, gradually increasing the speed, until the mixture is smooth. Pour into glasses and garnish the rim of each glass with a Strawberry Fan (page 212), if desired.

| | | | |
|---|---|---|---|
| Calories | 274 | Calcium | 66 mg |
| Calories from fat | 9 | Iron | 0.93 mg |
| Total fat | 1 g | Potassium | 866 mg |
| Carbohydrates | 69 g | Beta Carotene | 131 mcg |
| Protein | 3 g | Vitamin C | 166 mg |
| Fiber | 6 g | Folic Acid | 94 mcg |

# Peached Whale

*This whale of a smoothie is dedicated to serious peach lovers.*

### 2 SERVINGS

¾ cup peach nectar

1½ tablespoons honey

1½ cups peeled and diced peach (2 large peaches)

1 cup diced strawberries

1 cup sliced banana (1 large banana)

Place the nectar, honey, peach, strawberries, and banana in a blender, and mix on low speed until the mixture is blended. Continue mixing, gradually increasing the speed, until the mixture is smooth. Pour into glasses and garnish each with fresh mint, if desired.

| | | | |
|---|---|---|---|
| Calories | 247 | Calcium | 28 mg |
| Calories from fat | 7 | Iron | 0.93 mg |
| Total fat | 0.80 g | Potassium | 732 mg |
| Carbohydrates | 64 g | Beta Carotene | 506 mcg |
| Protein | 2 g | Magnesium | 43 mg |
| Fiber | 7 g | Vitamin C | 67 mg |

# Tropical Squeeze

*As you enjoy this delightful tropical fruit smoothie, imagine yourself on an island, where palm trees sway in the tropical breeze and the aroma of flowers brings thoughts of paradise.*

2 SERVINGS

¾ cup orange juice

1 tablespoon honey

1 cup peeled and diced mango (1 large mango)

1 cup diced pineapple (½ pineapple)

1 cup sliced banana (1 large banana)

¾ cup crushed ice

Place the juice, honey, mango, pineapple, banana, and ice in a blender and mix on low speed until the mixture is blended. Continue mixing, gradually increasing the speed, until the mixture is smooth. Pour into glasses and garnish the rim of each glass with a Pineapple, Orange, and Cherry Blossom (page 207), if desired.

| | | | |
|---|---|---|---|
| Calories | 235 | Calcium | 29 mg |
| Calories from fat | 10 | Iron | 0.86 mg |
| Total fat | 1 g | Potassium | 705 mg |
| Carbohydrates | 60 g | Beta Carotene | 2005 mcg |
| Protein | 2 g | Vitamin C | 88 mg |
| Fiber | 4 g | Folic Acid | 62 mcg |

# The Ultimate Fuzzy Navel Smoothie

*The term* fuzzy navel *refers to peach "fuzz" and a "navel" orange. The flavors blend as wonderfully as the words.*

### 2 SERVINGS

1 cup orange juice

1 ½ tablespoons honey

2 cups peeled and diced peach (2 large peaches)

1 cup sliced banana (1 large banana)

Place the juice, honey, peach, and banana in a blender, and mix on low speed until the mixture is blended. Continue mixing, gradually increasing the speed, until the mixture is smooth. Pour into glasses and garnish the rim of each glass with an Orange Wheel (page 199), if desired.

| | | | |
|---|---|---|---|
| Calories | 246 | Calcium | 28 mg |
| Calories from fat | 7 | Iron | 0.73 mg |
| Total fat | 0.76 g | Potassium | 888 mg |
| Carbohydrates | 62 g | Beta Carotene | 534 mcg |
| Protein | 3 g | Vitamin C | 80 mg |
| Fiber | 5 g | Folic Acid | 58 mcg |

# Vanna Banana

*You'll stop spinning your wheels and realize your good fortune when you taste the pleasing blend of strawberries and bananas in this classic smoothie.*

2 SERVINGS

1 cup orange juice

1 tablespoon honey

2 cups diced strawberries

2 cups sliced banana (2 large bananas)

2 to 3 teaspoons raspberry or strawberry preserves (optional)

Place the juice, honey, strawberries, banana, and optional preserves in a blender, and mix on low speed until the mixture is blended. Continue mixing, gradually increasing the speed, until the mixture is smooth. Pour into glasses and garnish the rim of each glass with a Strawberry Fan (page 212), if desired.

| | | | |
|---|---|---|---|
| Calories | 276 | Calcium | 47 mg |
| Calories from fat | 14 | Iron | 1 mg |
| Total fat | 2 g | Potassium | 1123 mg |
| Carbohydrates | 68 g | Beta Carotene | 145 mcg |
| Protein | 3 g | Magnesium | 74 mg |
| Fiber | 8 g | Vitamin C | 170 mg |

# Very Cherry (Not Contrary) Smoothie

*There is nothing contrary about this smoothie. Its pleasing flavor will always put you in a positive mood.*

2 SERVINGS

1 cup white grape juice

1 tablespoon honey

1½ cups stemmed and diced Bing cherries

1 cup peeled and diced papaya (1 large papaya)

1 cup sliced banana (1 large banana)

Place the juice, honey, cherries, papaya, and banana in a blender, and mix on low speed until the mixture is blended. Continue mixing, gradually increasing the speed, until the mixture is smooth. Pour into glasses and garnish the rim of each glass with a Lemon and Cranberry Twist (page 197), if desired.

| | | | |
|---|---|---|---|
| Calories | 284 | Calcium | 50 mg |
| Calories from fat | 14 | Iron | 1 mg |
| Total fat | 2 g | Potassium | 893 mg |
| Carbohydrates | 70 g | Beta Carotene | 204 mcg |
| Protein | 3 g | Vitamin C | 58 mg |
| Fiber | 6 g | Folic Acid | 49 mcg |

# *Watermelon Ecstasy*

*How much sweeter can it get than to enjoy a watermelon smoothie when the temperature is rising faster than the stock market?*

2 SERVINGS

1 cup pineapple juice

1 tablespoon honey

2 cups seeded and cubed watermelon (¼ melon)

1 ½ cups blueberries

Place the juice, honey, watermelon, and blueberries in a blender, and mix on low speed until the mixture is blended. Continue mixing, gradually increasing the speed, until the mixture is smooth. Pour into glasses and garnish each with Berries on a Skewer (page 169), if desired.

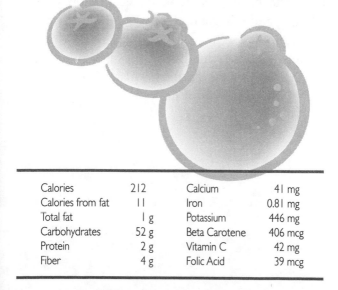

| Calories | 212 | Calcium | 41 mg |
|---|---|---|---|
| Calories from fat | 11 | Iron | 0.81 mg |
| Total fat | 1 g | Potassium | 446 mg |
| Carbohydrates | 52 g | Beta Carotene | 406 mcg |
| Protein | 2 g | Vitamin C | 42 mg |
| Fiber | 4 g | Folic Acid | 39 mcg |

# Where the Cheer and the Cantaloupe Play

*You'll never hear a discouraging word from friends or family when you rev up your blender to create this refreshing blend of unusual ingredients and sensational tastes.*

2 SERVINGS

8 pitted dates, diced*

1 cup peach nectar

1 tablespoon honey

2 cups diced cantaloupe (¼ cantaloupe)

2 cups sliced banana (2 large bananas)

Place the pureed dates with nectar, honey, cantaloupe, and banana in a blender, and mix on low speed until the mixture is blended. Continue mixing, gradually increasing the speed, until the mixture is smooth. Pour into glasses and garnish each with fresh mint, if desired.

| Calories | 385 | Calcium | 44 mg |
|---|---|---|---|
| Calories from fat | 12 | Iron | 1 mg |
| Total fat | 1 g | Potassium | 1360 mg |
| Carbohydrates | 99 g | Beta Carotene | 3311 mcg |
| Protein | 4 g | Magnesium | 78 mg |
| Fiber | 8 g | Vitamin C | 88 mg |

**\*To puree dates:** Combine the dates and ½ cup boiling water in a cup; set aside for 15 minutes. Cover the cup with plastic wrap, and refrigerate for several hours or until well chilled. When chilled, drain the dates. Combine the dates and peach nectar in the blender and puree until smooth.

# Who Wants to Be a Melon-aire?

*If you love cantaloupe, you won't have to phone a friend before giving your final answer to this delicious question.*

2 SERVINGS

¾ cup orange juice

1 tablespoon honey

2 cups diced cantaloupe (¼ cantaloupe)

1½ cups peeled and diced peach (2 large peaches)

½ cup lemon sorbet

1 cup crushed ice

Place the juice, honey, cantaloupe, peach, sorbet, and ice in a blender, and mix on low speed until the mixture is blended. Continue mixing, gradually increasing the speed, until the mixture is smooth. Pour into glasses and garnish the rim of each glass with a Lime Wheel (page 199), if desired.

| Calories | 255 | Calcium | 35 mg |
|---|---|---|---|
| Calories from fat | 7 | Iron | 0.71 mg |
| Total fat | 0.75 g | Potassium | 952 mg |
| Carbohydrates | 63 g | Beta Carotene | 3445 mcg |
| Protein | 3 g | Vitamin C | 126 mg |
| Fiber | 4 g | Folic Acid | 60 mcg |

# Yada Yada Pineapple Colada

*On days when it seems as if no one is listening . . . yada yada yada, enjoy this pineapple smoothie and leave your troubles behind.*

## 2 SERVINGS

1 cup light coconut milk

¼ cup orange juice

2 cups diced pineapple (1 pineapple)

2 cups sliced banana (2 large bananas)

Place the coconut milk, juice, pineapple, and banana in a blender, and mix on low speed the mixture is blended. Continue mixing, gradually increasing the speed, until the mixture is smooth. Pour into glasses and garnish the rim of each glass with a Pineapple Spear (page 208), if desired.

| | | | |
|---|---|---|---|
| Calories | 296 | Calcium | 23 mg |
| Calories from fat | 68 | Iron | 2 mg |
| Total fat | 8 g | Potassium | 831 mg |
| Carbohydrates | 62 g | Beta Carotene | 102 mcg |
| Protein | 4 g | Magnesium | 69 mg |
| Fiber | 6 g | Folic Acid | 54 mcg |

# CHAPTER 5

# SmooootHies!

## Dairy Can Be Merry

For many of us, nothing is more divine than a basic smoothie made with fruit juice and fruit. However, if you haven't tried a smoothie made with milk, yogurt, or ice cream, you are in for a real treat. The addition of any of these ingredients results in a smoothie with a creamier texture and a richer taste. Just as important, with this combination of ingredients, you can reap the health benefits of eating both fruit and dairy, each vital components of the food pyramid. Once you have enjoyed the taste of such smoothies as War and Peach, Takes Two to Mango, or Shaked-Pear in Love, you will be eager to sample all thirty-seven recipes in this chapter.

Just like you, the dairy items in your diet
have grown up. Forget that warm glass of milk
at bedtime, and enjoy one of these cool and refreshing creations.

# A One, and a Two, and a Three Fruit Smoothie

*You won't need champagne bubbles or an orchestra to sit back, relax, and enjoy this refreshing smoothie.*

### 2 SERVINGS

½ cup peach nectar

I tablespoon honey

¾ cup peeled and diced peach (I peach)

¾ cup sliced banana (I banana)

¾ cup raspberries

I cup vanilla fat-free frozen yogurt

½ cup vanilla lowfat yogurt

Place the nectar, honey, peach, banana, raspberries, and yogurts in a blender, and mix on low speed until the mixture is blended. Continue mixing, gradually increasing the speed, until the mixture is smooth. Pour into glasses and garnish each with Berries on a Skewer (page 169), if desired.

| | | | |
|---|---|---|---|
| Calories | 320 | Calcium | 225 mg |
| Calories from fat | 12 | Iron | I mg |
| Total fat | I g | Potassium | 773 mg |
| Carbohydrates | 72 g | Beta Carotene | 293 mcg |
| Protein | 9 g | Magnesium | 42 mg |
| Fiber | 6 g | Folic Acid | 32 mcg |

# Apricot Heaven

*The best time to make this smoothie is when fresh apricots are in season. I like to buy them in quantity and then freeze them to use in a variety of smoothies.*

### 2 SERVINGS

½ cup apricot nectar

½ cup lowfat milk

1 tablespoon honey

2 cups diced apricots (8 apricots)

1½ cups sliced banana (2 large bananas)

Place the nectar, milk, honey, apricots, and banana in a blender, and mix on low speed until the mixture is blended. Continue mixing, gradually increasing the speed, until the mixture is smooth. Pour into glasses and garnish each with a sprig of mint, if desired.

| | | | |
|---|---|---|---|
| Calories | 278 | Calcium | 101 mg |
| Calories from fat | 22 | Iron | 1 mg |
| Total fat | 2 g | Potassium | 1084 mg |
| Carbohydrates | 65 g | Beta Carotene | 2961 mcg |
| Protein | 6 g | Magnesium | 48 mg |
| Fiber | 7 g | Folic Acid | 36 mcg |

# Banana and the King

*"Yul" be humming "Shall We Dance" after you experience the tropical essence of this delightful smoothie.*

2 SERVINGS

1 cup pineapple juice

1 tablespoon honey

2 cups sliced banana (2 large bananas)

2 cups pineapple lowfat frozen yogurt

Place the juice, honey, banana, and yogurt in a blender, and mix on low speed until the mixture is blended. Continue mixing, gradually increasing the speed, until the mixture is smooth. Pour into glasses and garnish each by inserting a Pineapple Chip (page 205) upright in the smoothie, if desired.

| | | | |
|---|---|---|---|
| Calories | 444 | Calcium | 338 mg |
| Calories from fat | 31 | Iron | 0.98 mg |
| Total fat | 3 g | Potassium | 1160 mg |
| Carbohydrates | 98 g | Beta Carotene | 76 mcg |
| Protein | 11 g | Magnesium | 89 mg |
| Fiber | 4 g | Folic Acid | 77 mcg |

# Blackberry Blast

*Whenever fresh blackberries are in season, I look for new ways to use them in smoothies. This combination is the ultimate way to blend their flavor.*

2 SERVINGS

½ cup apple juice

I tablespoon honey

I cup blackberries

I cup peeled and diced apple (I large apple)

I cup sliced banana (I large banana)

I cup vanilla lowfat yogurt

Place the juice, honey, blackberries, apple, banana, and yogurt in a blender, and mix on low speed until the mixture is blended. Continue mixing, gradually increasing the speed, until the mixture is smooth. Pour into glasses and garnish each with Berries on a Skewer (page 169), if desired.

| | | | |
|---|---|---|---|
| Calories | 305 | Calcium | 246 mg |
| Calories from fat | 22 | Iron | 1 mg |
| Total fat | 2 g | Potassium | 849 mg |
| Carbohydrates | 68 g | Beta Carotene | 82 mcg |
| Protein | 8 g | Magnesium | 61 mg |
| Fiber | 7 g | Folic Acid | 53 mcg |

# Blushing Raspberry and Peach Smoothie

*Don't be embarrassed if you fall in love with this enticing combination of flavors.*

### 2 SERVINGS

½ cup peach nectar

1 tablespoon honey

1 cup peeled and diced peach (1 large peach)

1 cup raspberries

1 cup sliced banana (1 large banana)

1 cup peach lowfat frozen yogurt

Place the nectar, honey, peach, raspberries, banana, and yogurt in a blender, and mix on low speed until the mixture is blended. Continue mixing, gradually increasing the speed, until the mixture is smooth. Pour into glasses and garnish each with fresh mint, if desired.

| | | | |
|---|---|---|---|
| Calories | 303 | Calcium | 179 mg |
| Calories from fat | 19 | Iron | 0.91 mg |
| Total fat | 2 g | Potassium | 785 mg |
| Carbohydrates | 70 g | Beta Carotene | 364 mcg |
| Protein | 7 g | Magnesium | 56 mg |
| Fiber | 8 g | Folic Acid | 44 mcg |

# Caramel Apple on a Stick

*This delightful reminiscence of your childhood has all the ingredients of a caramel apple except that a straw replaces the wooden stick.*

### 2 SERVINGS

1 cup apple juice

1 tablespoon honey

3 cups peeled and diced apple (3 large apples)

1 cup vanilla fat-free frozen yogurt

1 tablespoon cinnamon

½ teaspoon nutmeg

3 tablespoons caramel topping (or more), to taste

Place the juice, honey, apple, yogurt, cinnamon, and nutmeg in a blender, and mix on low speed until the mixture is blended. Continue mixing, gradually increasing the speed, until the mixture is smooth. Divide half of the smoothie into two cocktail glasses (filling each halfway) and spoon some of the caramel topping over each serving. Pour the remaining smoothie over the caramel

| Calories | 373 | Calcium | 247 mg |
|---|---|---|---|
| Calories from fat | 11 | Iron | 2 mg |
| Total fat | 1 g | Potassium | 602 mg |
| Carbohydrates | 91 g | Beta Carotene | 40 mcg |
| Protein | 6 g | Magnesium | 33 mg |
| Fiber | 7 g | Folic Acid | 17 mcg |

topping and spoon a dollop of caramel over each. Garnish by inserting two Cinnamon-Coated Fusilli (page 187) upright in each smoothie, if desired.

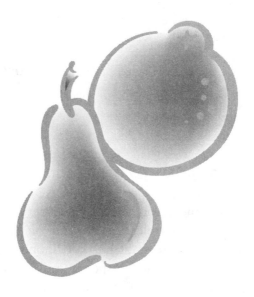

# Chai, Baby

*In many parts of the world, the word for "tea" is* chai *(rhymes with* pie*). The chai served in India is made with black tea, milk, a variety of spices, and a sweetener. This winning combination is a natural when blended with smoothie ingredients.*

### 2 SERVINGS

¾ cup chai tea (such as Celestial Seasonings' Bengal Spice), prepared with milk according to package instructions*

1 tablespoon honey

2 cups sliced banana (2 large bananas)

1 cup vanilla fat-free frozen yogurt

Refrigerate the prepared chai tea for 30 to 45 minutes or until cold.

Place the tea, honey, banana, and yogurt in a blender, and mix on low speed until the mixture is blended. Continue mixing, gradually increasing the speed, until the mixture is smooth. Pour into glasses and garnish each by inserting a cinnamon stick upright in the smoothie, if desired.

*If you have trouble finding chai tea, check your local health-food store.

| | | | |
|---|---|---|---|
| Calories | 326 | Calcium | 211 mg |
| Calories from fat | 14 | Iron | 0.59 mg |
| Total fat | 2 g | Potassium | 813 mg |
| Carbohydrates | 74 g | Beta Carotene | 72 mcg |
| Protein | 7 g | Magnesium | 60 mg |
| Fiber | 4 g | Folic Acid | 39 mcg |

# Cherry Bomb

*This cool indulgence explodes with the rich combination of cherry and strawberry flavors.*

2 SERVINGS

¾ cup lowfat milk

½ tablespoon honey

1 cup stemmed and seeded Bing cherries

1 cup sliced banana (1 large banana)

½ cup diced strawberries

1 cup vanilla fat-free frozen yogurt

Place the milk, honey, cherries, banana, strawberries, and yogurt in a blender, and mix on low speed until the mixture is blended. Continue mixing, gradually increasing the speed, until the mixture is smooth. Pour into glasses and garnish each with a Pineapple, Banana, and Cherry Charmer (page 204), if desired.

| | | | |
|---|---|---|---|
| Calories | 294 | Calcium | 290 mg |
| Calories from fat | 29 | Iron | 0.78 mg |
| Total fat | 3 g | Potassium | 899 mg |
| Carbohydrates | 61 g | Beta Carotene | 127 mcg |
| Protein | 10 g | Magnesium | 50 mg |
| Fiber | 4 g | Vitamin C | 36 mg |

# Cherry Springer

*You won't have to have a fistfight with your neighbor's boyfriend to get a taste of this knockout of a smoothie.*

### 2 SERVINGS

1 cup pineapple juice

1 tablespoon honey

2 cups stemmed and seeded Bing cherries

1 cup sliced banana (1 large banana)

1 cup black cherry lowfat frozen yogurt*

Place the juice, honey, cherries, banana, and yogurt in a blender, and mix on low speed the mixture is blended. Continue mixing, gradually increasing the speed, until the mixture is smooth. Pour into glasses and garnish each with a Lemon, Lime, and Cherry Boat (page 198), if desired.

*For a different taste sensation, try Ben & Jerry's Cherry Garcia lowfat frozen yogurt made with bits of chocolate.

| | | | | |
|---|---|---|---|---|
| Calories | 378 | Calcium | 20 mg |
| Calories from fat | 28 | Iron | 1 mg |
| Total fat | 3 g | Potassium | 991 mg |
| Carbohydrates | 86 g | Beta Carotene | 208 mcg |
| Protein | 7 g | Magnesium | 69 mg |
| Fiber | 5 g | Folic Acid | 59 mcg |

# Cinnamon Blueberry Calendar

*Why is this smoothie a calendar? It has lots of dates. Adding a touch of cinnamon to this interesting combination of blueberries and dates gives it just enough spice so that the flavors linger long after the first taste.*

## 2 SERVINGS

8 pitted dates, diced and pureed*

1 cup lowfat milk

1 tablespoon honey

1½ cups blueberries

1½ cups sliced banana (2 large bananas)

1 cup blueberry lowfat frozen yogurt

½ teaspoon cinnamon

Place the pureed dates with milk, honey, blueberries, banana, yogurt, and cinnamon in a blender, and mix on low speed until the mixture is blended. Continue mixing, gradually increasing the speed, until the mixture is smooth. Pour into glasses and garnish by inserting two Cinnamon-

| Calories | 456 | Calcium | 320 mg |
|---|---|---|---|
| Calories from fat | 44 | Iron | 1 mg |
| Total fat | 5 g | Potassium | 1169 mg |
| Carbohydrates | 100 g | Beta Carotene | 130 mcg |
| Protein | 11 g | Magnesium | 65 mg |
| Fiber | 8 g | Folic Acid | 42 mcg |

Coated Fusilli (page 187) upright in each smoothie, if desired.

**\*To puree dates:** Combine the dates and ½ cup boiling water in a cup; set aside for 15 minutes. Cover the cup with plastic wrap and refrigerate for several hours or until well chilled. When chilled, drain the dates. Combine the dates and milk in the blender and puree. Add the remaining ingredients and proceed accordingly.

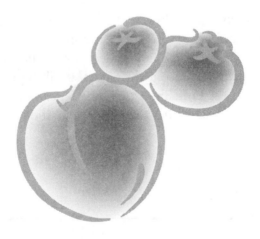

# Going Bananas over Cantaloupe

*This is no monkey business. Cantaloupe combined with banana yields a unique combination of flavors that is ideal for a frosty smoothie.*

### 2 SERVINGS

½ cup fresh orange juice

1 tablespoon honey

2 cups sliced banana (2 large bananas)

1½ cups diced cantaloupe (¼ cantaloupe)

1 cup vanilla lowfat yogurt

1 cup crushed ice

Place the juice, honey, banana, cantaloupe, yogurt, and ice in a blender, and mix on low speed until the mixture is blended. Continue mixing, gradually increasing the speed, until the mixture is smooth. Pour into glasses and garnish the rim of each glass with a slice of orange, if desired.

| | | | |
|---|---|---|---|
| Calories | 345 | Calcium | 239 mg |
| Calories from fat | 24 | Iron | 0.97 mg |
| Total fat | 3 g | Potassium | 1363 mg |
| Carbohydrates | 77 g | Beta Carotene | 2400 mcg |
| Protein | 9 g | Magnesium | 84 mg |
| Fiber | 5 g | Vitamin C | 96 mg |

# Heavenly Hawaiian

*The pineapple flavor of this refreshing smoothie is the next best thing to relaxing on the beach in Waikiki.*

### 2 SERVINGS

¾ cup pineapple juice

½ tablespoon honey

1 cup sliced banana (1 large banana)

1 cup diced pineapple (½ pineapple)

¾ cup raspberries

1 cup vanilla lowfat yogurt

Place the juice, honey, banana, pineapple, raspberries, and yogurt in a blender, and mix on low speed until the mixture is blended. Continue mixing, gradually increasing the speed, until the mixture is smooth. Pour into glasses and garnish each with a Pineapple, Orange, and Cherry Blossom (page 207), if desired.

| | | | |
|---|---|---|---|
| Calories | 303 | Calcium | 246 mg |
| Calories from fat | 23 | Iron | 1 mg |
| Total fat | 3 g | Potassium | 851 mg |
| Carbohydrates | 67 g | Beta Carotene | 66 mcg |
| Protein | 8 g | Magnesium | 73 mg |
| Fiber | 6 g | Folic Acid | 69 mcg |

# Honey, I Ate the Banana Smoothie

*You won't shrink from the task of making this smoothie over and over again once you taste this pleasingly sweet combination of honey and bananas together.*

## 2 SERVINGS

½ cup honey

¾ teaspoon vanilla extract

2 cups sliced banana (2 large bananas)

1½ cups vanilla lowfat yogurt

Place the honey, vanilla, banana, and yogurt in a blender, and mix on low speed until the mixture is blended. Continue mixing, gradually increasing the speed, until the mixture is smooth. Pour into glasses and garnish by inserting two Cinnamon-Coated Fusilli (page 187) upright in each smoothie, if desired.

| | | | |
|---|---|---|---|
| Calories | 557 | Calcium | 328 mg |
| Calories from fat | 27 | Iron | 0.95 mg |
| Total fat | 3 g | Potassium | 1043 mg |
| Carbohydrates | 131 g | Beta Carotene | 72 mcg |
| Protein | 11 g | Magnesium | 76 mg |
| Fiber | 4 g | Folic Acid | 50 mcg |

# Last Mango in Paris

*But hopefully, not the last one at your super-market. Mangoes are an ideal fruit to include in a smoothie. Their bold flavor, beautiful color, and soft flesh marry so well with most other fruits and dairy products that they are the ideal smoothie ingredient.*

## 2 SERVINGS

½ cup pineapple juice

1 tablespoon honey

2 cups peeled and diced mango (1 large mango)

1 cup vanilla fat-free yogurt

¾ cup crushed ice

Place the juice, honey, mango, yogurt, and ice in a blender, and mix on low speed until the mixture is blended. Continue mixing, gradually increasing the speed, until the mixture is smooth. Pour into glasses and garnish each with a Fruit Skewer (page 195), if desired.

| | | | |
|---|---|---|---|
| Calories | 286 | Calcium | 246 mg |
| Calories from fat | 6 | Iron | 0.53 mg |
| Total fat | 0.69 g | Potassium | 626 mg |
| Carbohydrates | 67 g | Beta Carotene | 3853 mcg |
| Protein | 7 g | Vitamin C | 53 mg |
| Fiber | 3 g | Folic Acid | 51 mcg |

# Leaping Pineapple Blizzard

*Even Annie would sing for this delightful pineapple smoothie—today, tomorrow, or any time.*

## 2 SERVINGS

¾ cup lowfat milk

1 tablespoon honey

2 cups cubed pineapple (1 pineapple)

1 cup tropical-flavored sherbet

1 cup crushed ice

Place the milk, honey, pineapple, sherbet, and ice in a blender, and mix on low speed until the mixture is blended. Continue mixing, gradually increasing the speed, until the mixture is smooth. Pour into glasses and garnish each with a Pineapple Spear (page 208), if desired.

| | | | |
|---|---|---|---|
| Calories | 294 | Calcium | 166 mg |
| Calories from fat | 41 | Iron | 0.76 mg |
| Total fat | 5 g | Potassium | 429 mg |
| Carbohydrates | 70 g | Magnesium | 30 mg |
| Protein | 5 g | Vitamin C | 37 mg |
| Fiber | 2 g | Vitamin D | 37 IU |

# Mango, Banana, and Cantaloupe Collider

*You won't need to notify your insurance company about this collision, but you can be assured that your own company will let you know how much they enjoy this refreshing treat.*

### 2 SERVINGS

¾ cup pineapple juice

1 tablespoon honey

1 cup peeled and diced mango (1 large mango)

1 cup sliced banana (1 large banana)

1 cup diced cantaloupe (⅛ cantaloupe)

1 cup banana lowfat frozen yogurt

Place the juice, honey, mango, banana, cantaloupe, and yogurt in a blender, and mix on low speed until the mixture is blended. Continue mixing, gradually increasing the speed, until the mixture is smooth. Pour into glasses and garnish each with Melon Balls on a Skewer (page 202), if desired.

| | | | | |
|---|---|---|---|---|
| Calories | 337 | Calcium | 192 mg |
| Calories from fat | 20 | Iron | 0.87 mg |
| Total fat | 2 g | Potassium | 1001 mg |
| Carbohydrates | 78 g | Beta Carotene | 3500 mcg |
| Protein | 7 g | Vitamin A | 598 mcg |
| Fiber | 4 g | Vitamin C | 74 mg |

# Mango Creamsicle Smoothie

*This is truly the next best thing to eating a cream-sicle on a stick. You can't help being in Good Humor after one taste of this delight.*

2 SERVINGS

1 cup orange juice

3 cups peeled and diced mango (3 large mangoes)

1 cup vanilla fat-free frozen yogurt

Place the juice, mango, and yogurt in a blender, and mix on low speed until the mixture is blended. Continue mixing, gradually increasing the speed, until the mixture is smooth. Pour into glasses and garnish the rim of each glass with an Orange Wheel (page 199), if desired.

| | | | |
|---|---|---|---|
| Calories | 312 | Calcium | 206 mg |
| Calories from fat | 10 | Iron | 0.65 mg |
| Total fat | 1 g | Potassium | 848 mg |
| Carbohydrates | 74 g | Beta Carotene | 5823 mcg |
| Protein | 7 g | Vitamin A | 989 mcg |
| Fiber | 5 g | Vitamin C | 131 mg |

# Mango...
# Jane and Boy Stay

*This pleasingly sweet smoothie will civilize your most primitive instincts. You may not be cruising from treetop to treetop, but you'll be swinging on your patio.*

2 SERVINGS

6 tablespoons apricot nectar

1 tablespoon honey

3 cups peeled and diced mango (3 large mangoes)

½ cup mango sorbet

½ cup vanilla lowfat yogurt

Place the nectar, honey, mango, sorbet, and yogurt in a blender, and mix on low speed until the mixture is blended. Continue mixing, gradually increasing the speed, until the mixture is smooth. Pour into glasses and garnish the rim of each glass with a slice of mango, if desired.

| | | | |
|---|---|---|---|
| Calories | 332 | Calcium | 136 mg |
| Calories from fat | 14 | Iron | 0.64 mg |
| Total fat | 2 g | Potassium | 579 mg |
| Carbohydrates | 81 g | Beta Carotene | 6147 mcg |
| Protein | 5 g | Vitamin A | 1196 mcg |
| Fiber | 5 g | Vitamin C | 75 mg |

# Mango Tango

*Shall we dance? This delicious smoothie will get your feet tapping and your hips swaying.*

2 SERVINGS

¼ cup orange juice

1 tablespoon honey

3 cups peeled and diced mango (3 large mangoes)

1 cup pineapple lowfat frozen yogurt

½ cup crushed ice

Place the juice, honey, mango, yogurt, and ice in a blender, and mix on low speed until the mixture is blended. Continue mixing, gradually increasing the speed, until the mixture is smooth. Pour into glasses and garnish each with a Fruit Skewer (page 195), if desired.

| | | | |
|---|---|---|---|
| Calories | 309 | Calcium | 182 mg |
| Calories from fat | 18 | Iron | 0.50 mg |
| Total fat | 2 g | Potassium | 650 mg |
| Carbohydrates | 72 g | Beta Carotene | 5788 mcg |
| Protein | 6 g | Vitamin A | 982 mcg |
| Fiber | 5 g | Vitamin C | 85 mg |

# Most Excellent Banana and Peach Smoothie

*The name of this smoothie says it all! Believe me, your enthusiasm will not "Wayne" when you taste this world-class creation.*

### 2 SERVINGS

¼ cup peach nectar

¼ cup orange juice

1 tablespoon honey

1 ½ cups sliced banana (2 large bananas)

1 cup peeled and diced peach (1 large peach)

1 cup vanilla lowfat yogurt

1 cup crushed ice

Place the nectar, juice, honey, banana, peach, yogurt and ice in a blender, and mix on low speed until the mixture is blended. Continue mixing, gradually increasing the speed, until the mixture is smooth. Pour into glasses and garnish each with an Orange, Lemon, and Cherry Combo (page 203), if desired.

| | | | |
|---|---|---|---|
| Calories | 308 | Calcium | 226 mg |
| Calories from fat | 20 | Iron | 0.69 mg |
| Total fat | 2 g | Potassium | 961 mg |
| Carbohydrates | 69 g | Beta Carotene | 331 mcg |
| Protein | 8 g | Magnesium | 64 mg |
| Fiber | 5 g | Folic Acid | 47 mcg |

# Oh My Papaya

*If you're into nostalgia, buy the record. If you're longing for great flavors, try this original cast production.*

2 SERVINGS

½ cup apple juice

1 tablespoon honey

1 cup peeled and diced papaya (1 large papaya)

1 cup sliced banana (1 large banana)

1 cup raspberries

1 cup vanilla fat-free frozen yogurt

Place the juice, honey, papaya, banana, raspberries, and yogurt in a blender, and mix on low speed until the mixture is blended. Continue mixing, gradually increasing the speed, until the mixture is smooth. Pour into glasses and garnish each by inserting an Apple Chip (page 167) upright in the smoothie, if desired.

| | | | |
|---|---|---|---|
| Calories | 283 | Calcium | 207 mg |
| Calories from fat | 9 | Iron | 1 mg |
| Total fat | 1 g | Potassium | 864 mg |
| Carbohydrates | 67 g | Beta Carotene | 95 mcg |
| Protein | 7 g | Vitamin C | 67 mg |
| Fiber | 7 g | Folic Acid | 67 mcg |

# Passion Fruit Hoot

*Combining two fruits and passion juice with fresh banana frozen yogurt is a real treat. If you only have vanilla yogurt on hand, the smoothie will still be delicious.*

2 SERVINGS

1 cup passion fruit nectar

1 tablespoon honey

1½ cups blueberries

1½ cups sliced banana (2 large bananas)

1 cup banana lowfat frozen yogurt

Place the nectar, honey, blueberries, banana, and yogurt in a blender, and mix on low speed until the mixture is blended. Continue mixing, gradually increasing the speed, until the mixture is smooth. Pour into glasses and garnish each with a Fruit Skewer (page 195), if desired.

| | | | |
|---|---|---|---|
| Calories | 381 | Calcium | 171 mg |
| Calories from fat | 21 | Iron | 0.79 mg |
| Total fat | 2 g | Potassium | 883 mg |
| Carbohydrates | 90 g | Beta Carotene | 119 mcg |
| Protein | 7 g | Magnesium | 62 mg |
| Fiber | 6 g | Vitamin A | 69 mcg |

# Peach and Pineapple Fling

*Thinking about one more fling? Try this wonderful fruit combination (or did you have something else in mind?).*

2 SERVINGS

1 cup pineapple juice

1½ cups peeled and diced peach (2 large peaches)

1½ cups diced pineapple (1 pineapple)

1 cup peach lowfat frozen yogurt

Place the juice, peach, pineapple, and yogurt in a blender, and mix on low speed until the mixture is blended. Continue mixing, gradually increasing the speed, until the mixture is smooth. Pour into glasses and garnish the rim of each glass with a slice of peach, if desired.

| | | | |
|---|---|---|---|
| Calories | 284 | Calcium | 189 mg |
| Calories from fat | 18 | Iron | 0.97 mg |
| Total fat | 2 g | Potassium | 747 mg |
| Carbohydrates | 64 g | Beta Carotene | 356 mcg |
| Protein | 6 g | Vitamin A | 85 mcg |
| Fiber | 4 g | Folic Acid | 55 mcg |

# Peach Blanket Bingo

*Join Frankie, Annette, and the other peach lovers for a rockin' good smoothie.*

### 2 SERVINGS

¾ cup peach nectar

½ tablespoon honey

1½ cups peeled and diced peach (2 large peaches)

1 cup peeled and diced papaya (1 large papaya)

1 cup peach lowfat frozen yogurt

Place the nectar, honey, peach, papaya, and yogurt in a blender, and mix on low speed until the mixture is blended. Continue mixing, gradually increasing the speed, until the mixture is smooth. Pour into glasses and garnish the rim of each glass with a Lime Wheel (page 199), if desired.

| | | | | |
|---|---|---|---|---|
| Calories | 250 | Calcium | 182 mg |
| Calories from fat | 14 | Iron | 0.48 mg |
| Total fat | 2 g | Potassium | 668 mg |
| Carbohydrates | 57 g | Beta Carotene | 491 mcg |
| Protein | 6 g | Vitamin A | 126 mcg |
| Fiber | 4 g | Vitamin C | 57 mg |

# Peter, Peter, Pumpkin Smoothie

*The best time of the year to serve this smoothie is during the months of October and November. Anything prepared then with pumpkins will put you in a festive mood.*

2 SERVINGS

1 cup lowfat milk

2 tablespoons honey

1 cup solid-packed pumpkin

1 cup sliced banana (1 large banana)

2 cups banana lowfat frozen yogurt

2 tablespoons dark brown sugar

1 teaspoon cinnamon

¼ teaspoon nutmeg

¼ teaspoon powdered ginger

Place the milk, honey, pumpkin, banana, yogurt, brown sugar, cinnamon, nutmeg, and ginger in a blender, and mix on low speed until the mixture is blended. Continue mixing, gradually in-

| | | | |
|---|---|---|---|
| Calories | 500 | Calcium | 515 mg |
| Calories from fat | 51 | Iron | 2 mg |
| Total fat | 6 g | Potassium | 963 mg |
| Carbohydrates | 102 g | Beta Carotene | 10621 mcg |
| Protein | 16 g | Magnesium | 57 mg |
| Fiber | 8 g | Vitamin A | 1901 mcg |

creasing the speed, until the mixture is smooth. Pour into glasses and garnish by inserting two Cinnamon-Coated Fusilli (page 187) upright in each smoothie, if desired.

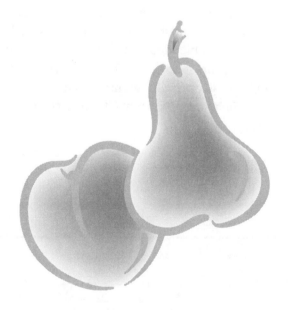

# Pineapple and Banana Fusion

*You don't have to be a nuclear scientist to understand why this fusion works so well. But just in case you are, the reason is:* $E = mc^2 + 2\pi r$.

## 2 SERVINGS

½ cup peach nectar

1 tablespoon honey

1 ¼ cups cubed pineapple (1 pineapple)

1 ¼ cups sliced banana (2 large bananas)

1 cup tropical-flavored sherbet

Place the nectar, honey, pineapple, banana, and sherbet in a blender, and mix on low speed until the mixture is blended. Continue mixing, gradually increasing the speed, until the mixture is smooth. Pour into glasses and garnish each with a Pineapple, Banana, and Cherry Charmer (page 204), if desired.

| | | | |
|---|---|---|---|
| Calories | 336 | Calcium | 70 mg |
| Calories from fat | 26 | Iron | 0.95 mg |
| Total fat | 3 g | Potassium | 606 mg |
| Carbohydrates | 81 g | Beta Carotene | 135 mcg |
| Protein | 3 g | Magnesium | 51 mg |
| Fiber | 4 g | Folic Acid | 34 mcg |

# Purple Passion Smoothie

*If purple is your favorite color and you have a passion for blueberries and blackberries, this smoothie is for you!*

2 SERVINGS

¾ cup cranberry juice

1 tablespoon honey

1 cup blueberries

1 cup blackberries

1 cup sliced banana (1 large banana)

1 cup Häagen-Dazs Vanilla Raspberry Swirl fat-free frozen yogurt or other raspberry swirl yogurt

Place the juice, honey, blueberries, blackberries, banana, and yogurt in a blender, and mix on low speed until the mixture is blended. Continue mixing, gradually increasing the speed, until the mixture is smooth. Pour into glasses and garnish each with a Fruit Skewer (page 195), if desired.

| | | | |
|---|---|---|---|
| Calories | 363 | Calcium | 135 mg |
| Calories from fat | 9 | Iron | 0.95 mg |
| Total fat | 1 g | Potassium | 525 mg |
| Carbohydrates | 87 g | Beta Carotene | 116 mcg |
| Protein | 6 g | Vitamin C | 65 mg |
| Fiber | 8 g | Folic Acid | 44 mcg |

# Rasanna Banana

*Enjoy this dazzling fusion of flavors any time of the day.*

### 2 SERVINGS

¾ cup pineapple juice

1 tablespoon honey

2 cups sliced banana (2 large bananas)

1 cup raspberries

1 cup banana lowfat frozen yogurt

Place the juice, honey, banana, raspberries, and yogurt in a blender, and mix on low speed until the mixture is blended. Continue mixing, gradually increasing the speed, until the mixture is smooth. Pour into glasses and garnish each with Berries on a Skewer (page 169), if desired.

| | | | |
|---|---|---|---|
| Calories | 355 | Calcium | 193 mg |
| Calories from fat | 22 | Iron | 1 mg |
| Total fat | 2 g | Potassium | 1015 mg |
| Carbohydrates | 82 g | Beta Carotene | 99 mcg |
| Protein | 7 g | Magnesium | 82 mg |
| Fiber | 8 g | Folic Acid | 76 mcg |

# *Razzamatazz Raspberry Smoothie*

*If you adore raspberries, don't look any further than this intensely flavorful delight.*

2 SERVINGS

6 tablespoons apple juice

1 tablespoon honey

1½ cups raspberries

1½ cups vanilla lowfat yogurt

1 cup raspberry sorbet

Place the juice, honey, raspberries, yogurt, and sorbet in a blender, and mix on low speed until the mixture is blended. Continue mixing, gradually increasing the speed, until the mixture is smooth. Pour into glasses and garnish each with Berries on a Skewer (page 169), if desired.

| | | | |
|---|---|---|---|
| Calories | 366 | Calcium | 338 mg |
| Calories from fat | 26 | Iron | 0.87 mg |
| Total fat | 3 g | Potassium | 663 mg |
| Carbohydrates | 77 g | Magnesium | 48 mg |
| Protein | 10 g | Vitamin C | 32 mg |
| Fiber | 6 g | Folic Acid | 44 mcg |

# Savannah Banana Smoothie

*The orange flavor from the juice and sherbet is re-freshingly apparent in this exceptional banana smoothie.*

2 SERVINGS

1 cup orange juice

½ cup lowfat milk

1 tablespoon honey

2 cups sliced banana (2 large bananas)

1 cup raspberry sorbet

Place the juice, milk, honey, banana, and sorbet in a blender, and mix on low speed until the mixture is blended. Continue mixing, gradually increasing the speed, until the mixture is smooth. Pour into glasses and garnish the rim of each glass with a slice of orange, if desired.

| | | | |
|---|---|---|---|
| Calories | 368 | Calcium | 91 mg |
| Calories from fat | 20 | Iron | 0.76 mg |
| Total fat | 2 g | Potassium | 1010 mg |
| Carbohydrates | 87 g | Beta Carotene | 118 mcg |
| Protein | 4 g | Vitamin A | 74 mcg |
| Fiber | 4 g | Vitamin C | 82 mg |

# Shaked-Pear in Love

*Get thee to the produce department! This smoothie was not only created for pear devotees but also for proof that when using fall fruit, smoothies can be enjoyed any time of the year.*

2 SERVINGS

½ cup pear nectar

2 tablespoons maple syrup

1 tablespoon honey

2 cups peeled and diced pear (2 large pears)

1 cup sliced banana (1 large banana)

1¼ cups banana lowfat frozen yogurt

½ teaspoon cinnamon

¼ teaspoon nutmeg

¼ teaspoon powdered ginger

Place the nectar, maple syrup, honey, pear, banana, yogurt, cinnamon, nutmeg, and ginger in a blender, and mix on low speed until the mixture

| | | | |
|---|---|---|---|
| Calories | 419 | Calcium | 239 mg |
| Calories from fat | 25 | Iron | 1 mg |
| Total fat | 3 g | Potassium | 810 mg |
| Carbohydrates | 98 g | Beta Carotene | 57 mcg |
| Protein | 7 g | Magnesium | 56 mg |
| Fiber | 7 g | Folic Acid | 40 mcg |

is blended. Continue mixing, gradually increasing the speed, until the mixture is smooth. Pour into glasses and garnish each with a Cinnamon Wonton Crisp (page 189), if desired.

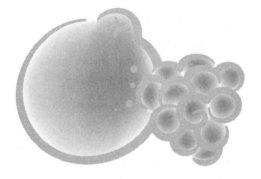

# Strawberry Starwhip

*If you live near a strawberry farm where you can pick your own fruit, take advantage of the opportunity to truly appreciate the strawberries' fresh flavors. If you can keep yourself from eating this bounty before you get home, the next best thing will be enjoying this strawberry creation.*

### 2 SERVINGS

I cup lowfat milk

¼ cup honey

2 cups diced strawberries

I cup vanilla lowfat yogurt

I cup crushed ice

Place the milk, honey, strawberries, yogurt, and ice in a blender, and mix on low speed until the mixture is blended. Continue mixing, gradually increasing the speed, until the mixture is smooth. Pour into glasses and garnish the rim of each glass with a Strawberry Fan (page 212), if desired.

| | | | |
|---|---|---|---|
| Calories | 348 | Calcium | 370 mg |
| Calories from fat | 42 | Iron | 0.89 mg |
| Total fat | 5 g | Potassium | //1 mg |
| Carbohydrates | 70 g | Vitamin A | 96 mcg |
| Protein | 11 g | Vitamin C | 95 mg |
| Fiber | 4 g | Vitamin D | 51 IU |

# Takes Two to Mango

*This delight was especially designed for mango lovers. If you're not one yet, try this addicting combination of mango-enhancing flavors, and you'll be converted.*

2 SERVINGS

¾ cup orange juice

1 tablespoon honey

½ cup peeled and diced mango (1 mango)

1½ cups peeled and diced peach (2 large peaches)

1 cup mango sorbet

¾ cup crushed ice

Place the juice, honey, mango, peach, sorbet, and ice in a blender, and mix on low speed until the mixture is blended. Continue mixing, gradually increasing the speed, until the mixture is smooth. Pour into glasses and garnish the rim of each glass with a slice of peach, if desired.

| | | | |
|---|---|---|---|
| Calories | 277 | Calcium | 26 mg |
| Calories from fat | 5 | Iron | 0.54 mg |
| Total fat | 0.53 g | Potassium | 507 mg |
| Carbohydrates | 69 g | Beta Carotene | 1336 mcg |
| Protein | 2 g | Vitamin A | 574 mcg |
| Fiber | 4 g | Vitamin C | 78 mg |

# The Chicago Berries

*That's right—Da Berries! I used my juicer to make fresh grape juice to add to this captivating blend of berries. Whether you use fresh or bottled juice, the result will be an NFL (Naturally Flavorful Liquid) all-star.*

2 SERVINGS

¾ cup grape juice

1 tablespoon honey

1 cup blackberries

1 cup raspberries

1½ cups vanilla lowfat yogurt

Place the juice, honey, blackberries, raspberries, and yogurt in a blender, and mix on low speed until the mixture is blended. Continue mixing, gradually increasing the speed, until the mixture is smooth. Pour into glasses and garnish each with Berries on a Skewer (page 169), if desired.

| | | | |
|---|---|---|---|
| Calories | 315 | Calcium | 360 mg |
| Calories from fat | 27 | Iron | 1 mg |
| Total fat | 3 g | Potassium | 768 mg |
| Carbohydrates | 65 g | Magnesium | 65 mg |
| Protein | 11 g | Vitamin C | 32 mg |
| Fiber | 8 g | Folic Acid | 62 mcg |

# The Three Berries

*Has someone been tasting your smoothie? You bet—everyone will want to taste this tempting celebration of berries.*

2 SERVINGS

¾ cup peach nectar

1½ tablespoons honey

¾ cup blueberries

¾ cup raspberries

¾ cup blackberries

1 cup blueberry lowfat frozen yogurt

½ cup raspberry sorbet

Place the nectar, honey, blueberries, raspberries, blackberries, yogurt, and sorbet in a blender, and mix on low speed until the mixture is blended. Continue mixing, gradually increasing the speed, until the mixture is smooth. Pour into glasses and garnish each with Berries on a Skewer (page 169), if desired.

| | | | |
|---|---|---|---|
| Calories | 336 | Calcium | 190 mg |
| Calories from fat | 18 | Iron | 0.98 mg |
| Total fat | 2 g | Potassium | 497 mg |
| Carbohydrates | 78 g | Beta Carotene | 194 mcg |
| Protein | 6 g | Vitamin A | 58 mcg |
| Fiber | 8 g | Folic Acid | 45 mcg |

# War and Peach

*You'll be "Russian" to tell your friends about this novel combination of ingredients. The word* peach *is often used to show admiration, and after tasting this smoothie, you'll appreciate why the term is attributed to this fruit.*

## 2 SERVINGS

6 tablespoons peach nectar

1 tablespoon honey

3 cups peeled and diced peach (3 large peaches)

½ cup mango sorbet

½ cup vanilla lowfat yogurt

½ cup crushed ice

Place the nectar, honey, peach, sorbet, yogurt, and ice in a blender, and mix on low speed until the mixture is blended. Continue mixing, gradually increasing the speed, until the mixture is smooth. Pour into glasses and garnish the rim of each glass with a slice of peach, if desired.

| | | | |
|---|---|---|---|
| Calories | 280 | Calcium | 123 mg |
| Calories from fat | 10 | Iron | 0.51 mg |
| Total fat | 1 g | Potassium | 661 mg |
| Carbohydrates | 67 g | Beta Carotene | 736 mcg |
| Protein | 5 g | Magnesium | 30 mg |
| Fiber | 6 g | Vitamin A | 321 mcg |

# World Wide Watermelon

*You can search the Web for most everything today, but the one thing it can't do electronically is mix up a batch of this tasty combination of watermelon and strawberries.*

## 2 SERVINGS

¾ cup peach nectar

1½ tablespoons honey

2 cups seeded and diced watermelon (¼ melon)

1 cup diced strawberries

1 cup peach lowfat frozen yogurt

Place the nectar, honey, watermelon, strawberries, and yogurt in a blender, and mix on low speed until the mixture is blended. Continue mixing, gradually increasing the speed, until the mixture is smooth. Pour into glasses and garnish each with a Fruit Skewer (page 195), if desired.

| | | | |
|---|---|---|---|
| Calories | 274 | Calcium | 183 mg |
| Calories from fat | 21 | Iron | 0.89 mg |
| Total fat | 2 g | Potassium | 556 mg |
| Carbohydrates | 61 g | Beta Carotene | 468 mcg |
| Protein | 6 g | Vitamin A | 96 mcg |
| Fiber | 3 g | Vitamin C | 67 mg |

# CHAPTER 6

# $R_X$ Smoothies

Drink to Your Health

*A*s inherently healthful as smoothies are, they should not be thought of as a total meal replacement. However, when protein powders or other meal supplements are blended into a smoothie, you can create an instant meal in no time. In addition, smoothies can be nutritionally enhanced with the addition of one or more healthful supplements, such as herbs and extracts. These health-enhancing boosters are reputed to provide a variety of benefits, including enhancing your energy, improving your memory, protecting against colds, and helping to relieve stress. If you are looking for ways to include more soybean products in your diet, you need look no further than your blender. Although several of the recipes included in this chapter suggest using frozen yogurt, don't hesitate to substitute your favorite soybean product instead. When soy milk or soy yogurt is combined with other smoothie ingredients, they not only add flavor but at the same time greatly enhance a smoothie's health benefits.

In this chapter, you will be delighted to discover over twenty recipes designed to appeal to the most health-conscious among us, such as Peach Boys, Happily Ever Apple, and Zany, Brainy Gingko Fruit Smoothie. A smoothie can be prepared with almost any fruit, and when combined with your favorite soybean product, supplement, or herb, the end result will always be a sensationally healthful and delicious treat.

# All Powered-Up Smoothie

*If energy and excitement are what you need in the morning, start the day with this outrageously tasty smoothie that packs a powerful punch!*

### 2 SERVINGS

¾ cup apple juice

1 tablespoon honey

1 cup sliced banana (1 large banana)

1 cup diced strawberries

1 cup diced pineapple (½ pineapple)

1 cup vanilla fat-free frozen yogurt

1 to 3 tablespoons natural or vanilla protein powder, or according to specific brand label recommendations

1½ to 2 tablespoons raspberry preserves, or to taste

Place the juice, honey, banana, strawberries, pineapple, yogurt, protein powder, and raspberry preserves in a blender, and mix on low speed until the mixture is blended. Continue mixing, gradually increasing the speed, until the mixture is smooth. Pour into glasses and garnish each with a Pineapple Spear (page 208), if desired.

| | | | |
|---|---|---|---|
| Calories | 359 | Calcium | 216 mg |
| Calories from fat | 13 | Iron | 3 mg |
| Total fat | 1 g | Potassium | 885 mg |
| Carbohydrates | 83 g | Magnesium | 62 mg |
| Protein | 9 g | Vitamin C | 67 mg |
| Fiber | 5 g | Folic Acid | 56 mcg |

# *Banana Bliss*

*What can be more blissful than indulging in a smoothie that not only is good for you but tastes good, too?*

## 2 SERVINGS

½ cup apple cider

1 tablespoon honey

¼ teaspoon vanilla extract

1½ cups sliced banana (2 large bananas)

1 cup raspberries

1 cup blueberries

2 cartons (6 ounces each) banana-strawberry
    soy yogurt

½ teaspoon cinnamon

Place the cider, honey, vanilla, banana, raspberries, blueberries, yogurt, and cinnamon in a blender, and mix on low speed until the mixture is blended. Continue mixing, gradually increasing the speed, until the mixture is smooth. Pour into glasses and garnish each by inserting a cinnamon stick upright in the smoothie, if desired.

| | | | |
|---|---|---|---|
| Calories | 365 | Calcium | 235 mg |
| Calories from fat | 29 | Iron | 3 mg |
| Total fat | 3 g | Potassium | 680 mg |
| Carbohydrates | 82 g | Beta Carotene | 123 mcg |
| Protein | 7 g | Magnesium | 50 mg |
| Fiber | 9 g | Folic Acid | 43 mcg |

# Bee Healthy Raspberry Smoothie

*Raspberries, bananas, soy milk, and bee pollen combined into a smoothie become a satisfying and healthful meal or treat.*

2 SERVINGS

1 cup vanilla soy milk

1 tablespoon honey

1½ cups raspberries

1½ cups sliced banana (2 large bananas)

1 cup raspberry fat-free frozen yogurt

1 tablespoon bee pollen, or according to specific brand label recommendations

Place the soy milk, honey, raspberries, banana, yogurt, and bee pollen in a blender, and mix on low speed until the mixture is blended. Continue mixing, gradually increasing the speed, until the mixture is smooth. Pour into glasses and garnish each with Berries on a Skewer (page 169), if desired.

| | | | |
|---|---|---|---|
| Calories | 382 | Calcium | 238 mg |
| Calories from fat | 39 | Iron | 2 mg |
| Total fat | 4 g | Potassium | 918 mg |
| Carbohydrates | 80 g | Beta Carotene | 90 mcg |
| Protein | 11 g | Magnesium | 67 mg |
| Fiber | 9 g | Folic Acid | 56 mcg |

# Bee Pollen Power Plant

*If a jolt of energy is what you are looking for, this smoothie will get you buzzing!*

### 2 SERVINGS

½ cup lowfat milk

2 tablespoons honey

1 cup diced pineapple (½ pineapple)

1 cup sliced banana (1 large banana)

1 cup banana lowfat frozen yogurt

1 to 3 tablespoons natural or vanilla protein powder, or according to specific brand label recommendations

½ tablespoon brewers yeast, or according to specific brand label recommendations

½ tablespoon bee pollen, or according to specific brand label recommendations

Place the milk, honey, pineapple, banana, yogurt, protein powder, brewers yeast, and bee pollen in a blender, and mix on low speed until the mixture is

| | | | |
|---|---|---|---|
| Calories | 335 | Calcium | 258 mg |
| Calories from fat | 32 | Iron | 3 mg |
| Total fat | 4 g | Potassium | 754 mg |
| Carbohydrates | 69 g | Magnesium | 55 mg |
| Protein | 11 g | Vitamin A | 58 mcg |
| Fiber | 4 g | Folic Acid | 119 mcg |

blended. Continue mixing, gradually increasing the speed, until the mixture is smooth. Pour into glasses and garnish each with a Pineapple, Banana, and Cherry Charmer (page 204), if desired.

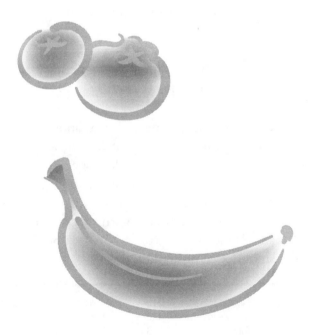

# Happily Ever Apple

*Once you have tasted this smoothie, you will be in a state of bliss; if not forever, at least for the rest of the day.*

### 2 SERVINGS

½ cup orange juice

1 tablespoon honey

2 teaspoons vanilla extract

1½ cups peeled and diced apple (2 large apples)

1½ cups sliced banana (2 large bananas)

1 cup banana lowfat frozen yogurt

½ cup wheat germ

3 tablespoons reduced-fat peanut butter

1 teaspoon cinnamon

Place the juice, honey, vanilla, apple, banana, yogurt, wheat germ, peanut butter, and cinnamon in a blender, and mix on low speed until the mixture is blended. Continue mixing, gradually increasing the speed, until the mixture is smooth. Pour into glasses and garnish each by inserting an Apple Chip (page 167) upright in the smoothie, if desired.

| Calories | 555 | Calcium | 209 mg |
|---|---|---|---|
| Calories from fat | 118 | Iron | 3 mg |
| Total fat | 13 g | Potassium | 1307 mg |
| Carbohydrates | 97 g | Magnesium | 128 mg |
| Protein | 20 g | Vitamin C | 47 mg |
| Fiber | 11 g | Folic Acid | 133 mcg |

# Havana Banana Energizer

*Like its bunny namesake, the lush tropical flavor of this smoothie just keeps going and going and going . . .*

2 SERVINGS

⅔ cup apple cider

1 tablespoon honey

2 cups sliced banana (2 large bananas)

1 cup raspberries

1 cup raspberry sorbet

½ tablespoon raspberry preserves

Ginseng, according to specific brand label recommendations

Place the cider, honey, banana, raspberries, sorbet, preserves, and ginseng in a blender, and mix on low speed until the mixture is blended. Continue mixing, gradually increasing the speed, until the mixture is smooth. Pour into glasses and garnish each glass with Berries on a Skewer (page 169), if desired.

| | | | |
|---|---|---|---|
| Calories | 358 | Calcium | 28 mg |
| Calories from fat | 10 | Iron | 1 mg |
| Total fat | 1 g | Potassium | 847 mg |
| Carbohydrates | 90 g | Beta Carotene | 96 mcg |
| Protein | 2 g | Magnesium | 57 mg |
| Fiber | 8 g | Folic Acid | 45 mcg |

# *Ivana Banana*

*A definite trump card that towers over most average smoothies. You won't let yourself be separated from this banana, strawberry, and peanut butter creation for any amount of money.*

### 2 SERVINGS

I cup vanilla soy milk

I tablespoon honey

1½ cups sliced banana (2 large bananas)

1½ cups diced strawberries

½ cup reduced-fat peanut butter

Place the soy milk, honey, banana, strawberries, and peanut butter in a blender, and mix on low speed until mixture is blended. Continue mixing, gradually increasing the speed, until the mixture is smooth. Pour into glasses and garnish the rim of each glass with a Strawberry Fan (page 212), if desired.

| | | | |
|---|---|---|---|
| Calories | 593 | Calcium | 91 mg |
| Calories from fat | 229 | Iron | 3 mg |
| Total fat | 25 g | Potassium | 1222 mg |
| Carbohydrates | 78 g | Beta Carotene | 74 mcg |
| Protein | 23 g | Magnesium | 45 mg |
| Fiber | 10 g | Vitamin C | 81 mg |

# Mango Magic

*Making smoothies with soy yogurt is a magically delicious way to add this important food to your diet.*

2 SERVINGS

1 cup orange juice

1 tablespoon honey

¼ teaspoon vanilla extract

1 ¼ cups peeled and diced mango (2 large mangoes)

1 ¼ cups sliced banana (2 large bananas)

1 ¼ cups diced pineapple (1 pineapple)

2 cartons (6 ounces each) apricot-mango soy yogurt

Place the juice, honey, vanilla, mango, banana, pineapple, and yogurt in a blender, and mix on low speed until mixture is blended. Continue mixing, gradually increasing the speed, until the mixture is smooth. Pour into glasses and garnish each with a Pineapple, Banana, and Cherry Charmer (page 204) if desired.

| | | | |
|---|---|---|---|
| Calories | 420 | Calcium | 286 mg |
| Calories from fat | 30 | Iron | 3 mg |
| Total fat | 3 g | Potassium | 896 mg |
| Carbohydrates | 96 g | Beta Carotene | 2509 mcg |
| Protein | 8 g | Magnesium | 64 mg |
| Fiber | 6 g | Folic Acid | 80 mcg |

# Oat Faithful Banana and Peanut Butter Blast

*Forget about old-fashioned oatmeal! There is no better way to start the morning than with this energizing smoothie made with bananas, oats, and peanut butter.*

### 2 SERVINGS

¾ cup lowfat milk

½ teaspoon vanilla extract

3 cups sliced banana (3 large bananas)

3 tablespoons reduced-fat peanut butter

1½ tablespoons oat bran

½ teaspoon cinnamon

Place the milk, vanilla, banana, peanut butter, oat bran, and cinnamon in a blender, and mix on low speed until the mixture is blended. Continue mixing, gradually increasing the speed, until the mixture is smooth. Pour into glasses and garnish each by inserting a cinnamon stick upright in the smoothie, if desired.

| | | | |
|---|---|---|---|
| Calories | 358 | Calcium | 132 mg |
| Calories from fat | 100 | Iron | 2 mg |
| Total fat | 11 g | Potassium | 1098 mg |
| Carbohydrates | 60 g | Beta Carotene | 91 mcg |
| Protein | 12 g | Magnesium | 65 mg |
| Fiber | 7 g | Vitamin A | 71 mcg |

# Peach Boys

*Whether you're surfing the waves or the Internet, you will find it hard to resist this tempting smoothie.*

### 2 SERVINGS

1 cup peach nectar

1 tablespoon honey

1½ cups peeled and diced peach (2 large peaches)

1 cup sliced banana (1 large banana)

1½ cups peach lowfat frozen yogurt

2 tablespoons flaxseed oil, or according to specific brand label recommendations

Place the nectar, honey, peach, banana, yogurt, and flaxseed oil in a blender, and mix on low speed until the mixture is blended. Continue mixing, gradually increasing the speed, until the mixture is smooth. Pour into glasses and garnish each with a Fruit Skewer (page 195), if desired.

| | | | |
|---|---|---|---|
| Calories | 495 | Calcium | 248 mg |
| Calories from fat | 144 | Iron | 0.77 mg |
| Total fat | 16 g | Potassium | 898 mg |
| Carbohydrates | 85 g | Beta Carotene | 532 mcg |
| Protein | 9 g | Magnesium | 58 mg |
| Fiber | 5 g | Vitamin A | 127 mcg |

# Peachy Keen Smoothie

*This smoothie tastes just peachy when you use fruit that is at the height of ripeness.*

2 SERVINGS

1 cup vanilla soy milk

½ cup peach nectar

1 tablespoon honey

3 cups peeled and diced peach (3 large peaches)

½ cup sliced banana (1 banana)

1 cup vanilla fat-free frozen yogurt

1 cup crushed ice

Place the soy milk, nectar, honey, peach, banana, yogurt, and ice in a blender, and mix on low speed until the mixture is blended. Continue mixing, gradually increasing the speed, until the mixture is smooth. Pour into glasses and garnish each with a Fruit Skewer (page 195), if desired.

| | | | |
|---|---|---|---|
| Calories | 400 | Calcium | 226 mg |
| Calories from fat | 32 | Iron | 1 mg |
| Total fat | 4 g | Potassium | 1001 mg |
| Carbohydrates | 87 g | Beta Carotene | 774 mcg |
| Protein | 11 g | Magnesium | 47 mg |
| Fiber | 6 g | Vitamin A | 159 mcg |

# Peanut Butter and Banana Avalanche

*Who doesn't love peanut butter? Now you can enjoy it in a nutritious smoothie without the guilt.*

2 SERVINGS

1 cup vanilla soy milk

1 tablespoon honey

2½ cups sliced banana (3 large bananas)

1 cup vanilla fat-free frozen yogurt

6 tablespoons reduced-fat peanut butter

1 tablespoon chocolate fudge sauce

1 tablespoon lecithin, or according to specific brand label recommendations

Place the soy milk, honey, banana, yogurt, peanut butter, fudge sauce, and lecithin in a blender, and mix on low speed until the mixture is blended. Continue mixing, gradually increasing the speed, until the mixture is smooth. Pour into glasses and garnish each by inserting a Crisp Banana Wafer (page 191) upright in the smoothie, if desired.

| | | | |
|---|---|---|---|
| Calories | 728 | Calcium | 247 mg |
| Calories from fat | 251 | Iron | 2 mg |
| Total fat | 28 g | Potassium | 1450 mg |
| Carbohydrates | 107 g | Beta Carotene | 90 mcg |
| Protein | 24 g | Magnesium | 76 mg |
| Fiber | 8 g | Folic Acid | 47 mcg |

# *Please Take the Kiwi to My Heart*

*You'll fall in love with this kiwi creation.*

### 2 SERVINGS

1 ½ cups pineapple juice

2 tablespoons honey

2 cups peeled and diced kiwi (12 kiwi)

1 cup sliced banana (1 large banana)

1 cup banana lowfat frozen yogurt

2 tablespoons flaxseed oil, or according to specific brand label recommendations

Place the juice, honey, kiwi, banana, yogurt, and flaxseed oil in a blender, and mix on low speed until the mixture is blended. Continue mixing, gradually increasing the speed, until the mixture is smooth. Pour into glasses and garnish the rim of each glass with a slice of kiwi, if desired.

| | | | |
|---|---|---|---|
| Calories | 568 | Calcium | 237 mg |
| Calories from fat | 145 | Iron | 2 mg |
| Total fat | 16 g | Potassium | 1343 mg |
| Carbohydrates | 106 g | Beta Carotene | 233 mcg |
| Protein | 8 g | Vitamin C | 201 mg |
| Fiber | 8 g | Folic Acid | 135 mcg |

# Purple Pleasure

*The color of the blueberries makes this delicious smoothie a rich purple, but the intense flavors of the other fruit will be savored with every sip.*

2 SERVINGS

½ cup vanilla soy milk

1 tablespoon honey

1 cup sliced banana (1 large banana)

1 cup raspberries

1 cup blueberries

1 cup vanilla fat-free frozen yogurt

½ cup strawberry sorbet

Place the soy milk, honey, banana, raspberries, blueberries, yogurt, and sorbet in a blender, and mix on low speed until the mixture is blended. Continue mixing, gradually increasing the speed, until the mixture is smooth. Pour into glasses and garnish each with Berries on a Skewer (page 169), if desired.

| | | | |
|---|---|---|---|
| Calories | 382 | Calcium | 214 mg |
| Calories from fat | 25 | Iron | 1 mg |
| Total fat | 3 g | Potassium | 727 mg |
| Carbohydrates | 86 g | Beta Carotene | 103 mcg |
| Protein | 9 g | Magnesium | 53 mg |
| Fiber | 9 g | Folic Acid | 45 mcg |

# Raspberry Ginseng Generator

*This smoothie will electrify you with that extra pep you need to get through the day.*

### 2 SERVINGS

¾ cup apple cider

1 tablespoon honey

1½ cups diced cantaloupe (¼ cantaloupe)

1½ cups diced raspberries

1 cup Häagen-Dazs Vanilla Raspberry Swirl fat-free frozen yogurt, or other yogurt

Ginseng to taste, or according to specific brand label recommendations

Place the cider, honey, cantaloupe, raspberries, yogurt, and ginseng in a blender, and mix on low speed until the mixture is blended. Continue mixing, gradually increasing the speed, until the mixture is smooth. Pour into glasses and garnish each with Melon Balls on a Skewer (page 202), if desired.

| | | | |
|---|---|---|---|
| Calories | 284 | Calcium | 139 mg |
| Calories from fat | 8 | Iron | 1 mg |
| Total fat | 0.93 g | Potassium | 605 mg |
| Carbohydrates | 66 g | Beta Carotene | 2340 mcg |
| Protein | 6 g | Vitamin A | 398 mcg |
| Fiber | 7 g | Vitamin C | 74 mg |

# Real Honey in the Bank

*This recipe will definitely generate a lot of interest. You can expect a monthly statement of delight from family and friends who try it.*

## 2 SERVINGS

½ cup vanilla soy milk

½ cup honey

¾ teaspoon vanilla extract

2½ cups sliced banana (3 large bananas)

1½ cups vanilla fat-free frozen yogurt

1 cup vanilla soy yogurt

Place the soy milk, honey, vanilla, banana, and yogurts in a blender, and mix on low speed until the mixture is blended. Continue mixing, gradually increasing the speed, until the mixture is smooth. Pour into glasses and garnish each by inserting a Crisp Banana Wafer (page 191) upright in the smoothie, if desired.

| | | | |
|---|---|---|---|
| Calories | 662 | Calcium | 371 mg |
| Calories from fat | 30 | Iron | 2 mg |
| Total fat | 3 g | Potassium | 1163 mg |
| Carbohydrates | 155 g | Beta Carotene | 90 mcg |
| Protein | 13 g | Magnesium | 80 mg |
| Fiber | 5 g | Folic Acid | 53 mcg |

# Soy Wonder

*You will be amazed that a smoothie could be so sinfully delicious and healthful at the same time.*

2 SERVINGS

¾ cup vanilla soy milk

½ cup apple juice

1 tablespoon honey

1 cup blueberries

1 cup sliced banana (1 large banana)

1 cup diced strawberries

1 cup vanilla fat-free frozen yogurt

½ cup strawberry sorbet

Place the soy milk, juice, honey, blueberries, banana, strawberries, yogurt, and sorbet in a blender, and mix on low speed until the mixture is blended. Continue mixing, gradually increasing the speed, until the mixture is smooth. Pour into glasses and garnish the rim of each glass with a Strawberry Fan (page 212), if desired.

| | | | |
|---|---|---|---|
| Calories | 429 | Calcium | 226 mg |
| Calories from fat | 32 | Iron | 1 mg |
| Total fat | 4 g | Potassium | 872 mg |
| Carbohydrates | 95 g | Beta Carotene | 93 mcg |
| Protein | 9 g | Magnesium | 52 mg |
| Fiber | 6 g | Vitamin C | 72 mg |

# Strawberried Treasure

*Yo ho ho and a bottle of fun! Strike your colors and sail into breakfast ecstasy with this nutritious smoothie.*

### 2 SERVINGS

2 cups vanilla soy milk

2 cups diced strawberries

2 cups sliced banana (2 large bananas)

2 packets Strawberry Crème Instant Breakfast

Place the soy milk, strawberries, banana, and instant breakfast in a blender, and mix on low speed until the mixture is blended. Continue mixing, gradually increasing the speed, until the mixture is smooth. Pour into glasses and garnish the rim of each glass with a Strawberry Fan (page 212), if desired.

| | | | |
|---|---|---|---|
| Calories | 508 | Calcium | 462 mg |
| Calories from fat | 66 | Iron | 6 mg |
| Total fat | 7 g | Potassium | 1330 mg |
| Carbohydrates | 102 g | Magnesium | 140 mg |
| Protein | 14 g | Vitamin A | 544 mcg |
| Fiber | 7 g | Folic Acid | 158 mcg |

# Strawberry and Banana Twister

*This smoothie disproves the theory that "anything that is good for you, can't taste good!"*

### 2 SERVINGS

1 cup vanilla soy milk

½ cup orange juice

1 tablespoon honey

1½ cups strawberries

1½ cups sliced banana (2 large bananas)

2 cartons (6 ounces each) strawberry-banana
  soy yogurt

Place the soy milk, juice, honey, strawberries, banana, and yogurt in a blender, and mix on low speed until the mixture is blended. Continue mixing, gradually increasing the speed, until the mixture is smooth. Pour into glasses and garnish each with a Fruit Skewer (page 195), if desired.

| | | | |
|---|---|---|---|
| Calories | 425 | Calcium | 271 mg |
| Calories from fat | 55 | Iron | 3 mg |
| Total fat | 6 g | Potassium | 887 mg |
| Carbohydrates | 87 g | Beta Carotene | 97 mcg |
| Protein | 11 g | Vitamin C | 115 mg |
| Fiber | 6 g | Folic Acid | 63 mcg |

# Strawberry, Banana, and Blueberry Banner

*This deliciously nutritious smoothie is a salute to the red, white, and blue!*

## 2 SERVINGS

¾ cup apple cider

1 tablespoon honey

1 cup strawberries

1 cup blueberries

1 cup sliced banana (1 large banana)

1 cup banana lowfat frozen yogurt

1 tablespoon lecithin, or according to specific brand label recommendations

Place the cider, honey, strawberries, blueberries, banana, yogurt, and lecithin in a blender, and mix on low speed until the mixture is blended. Continue mixing, gradually increasing the speed, until the mixture is smooth. Pour into glasses and garnish each by inserting an Apple Chip (page 167) upright in the smoothie, if desired.

| | | | |
|---|---|---|---|
| Calories | 360 | Calcium | 180 mg |
| Calories from fat | 82 | Iron | 1 mg |
| Total fat | 9 g | Potassium | 803 mg |
| Carbohydrates | 71 g | Beta Carotene | 93 mcg |
| Protein | 6 g | Magnesium | 51 mg |
| Fiber | 6 g | Vitamin C | 65 mg |

# Zany, Brainy Gingko Fruit Smoothie

*Get smart! Try this refreshing smoothie made with gingko—you'll never forget the recipe.*

2 SERVINGS

¾ cup apple cider

1 tablespoon honey

2 cups sliced banana (2 large bananas)

2 cups peeled and diced peach (2 large peaches)

1 cup peach lowfat frozen yogurt

Gingko biloba to taste, or according to specific brand label recommendations

Place the cider, honey, banana, peach, yogurt, and gingko in a blender, and mix on low speed until the mixture is blended. Continue mixing, gradually increasing the speed, until the mixture is smooth. Pour into glasses and garnish each with a Fruit Skewer (page 195), if desired.

| | | | |
|---|---|---|---|
| Calories | 385 | Calcium | 178 mg |
| Calories from fat | 20 | Iron | 1 mg |
| Total fat | 2 g | Potassium | 1232 mg |
| Carbohydrates | 91 g | Beta Carotene | 524 mcg |
| Protein | 7 g | Magnesium | 73 mg |
| Fiber | 7 g | Vitamin A | 117 mcg |

# CHAPTER 7

# Outrageously Decadent

Indulgence in a Glass

The overwhelming popularity of smoothies as a meal replacement, quick snack, or way to reduce dietary fat and calories cannot be disputed. But if you are looking for an occasional splurge, these versatile creations can also be made to order for that special indulgence. Smoothies can quickly be transformed into deliciously rich and delectable offerings that include such naughty ingredients as chocolate fudge, ice cream, cookies, and more. Most of the smoothies in this chapter incorporate fruit, and although they may be richer than usual, you will still reap the health benefits of including fruit and dairy products in your diet. But mostly, these smoothies are meant to be fun and enjoyed when a special treat is in order. Let your hair down and indulge in any of the recipes found in this chapter, such as Peanut Butter Decadence or The Pear Essentials. You'll find yourself counting the days until the next special occasion.

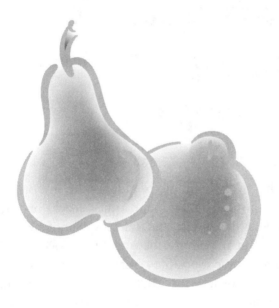

# Banana Boogie

*This smoothie will take you back to the good old days of malts, shakes, and rock and roll. So sidle up to the soda fountain and enjoy!*

2 SERVINGS

½ cup lowfat milk

1 ½ tablespoons honey

1 teaspoon vanilla extract

2 cups sliced banana (2 large bananas)

1 cup banana lowfat frozen yogurt

1 tablespoon light rum (optional)

Place the milk, honey, vanilla, banana, yogurt, and optional rum in a blender, and mix on low speed until the mixture is blended. Continue to mix, gradually increasing the speed, until the mixture is smooth. Pour into cocktail glasses and garnish each by inserting a Pirouette cookie (page 209) upright in the smoothie, if desired.

| | | | |
|---|---|---|---|
| Calories | 343 | Calcium | 231 mg |
| Calories from fat | 29 | Iron | 0.62 mg |
| Total fat | 3 g | Potassium | 905 mg |
| Carbohydrates | 70 g | Beta Carotene | 72 mcg |
| Protein | 8 g | Magnesium | 59 mg |
| Fiber | 4 g | Vitamin A | 63 mcg |

# The Big Banana Chill

*Once you have tasted this deliciously rich smoothie, you won't be able to stop telling your friends about it.*

2 SERVINGS

¼ cup lowfat milk

1 cup sliced banana (1 large banana)

1½ cups chocolate or vanilla ice cream

¼ cup peanut butter

3 tablespoons chocolate malted milk powder

Place the milk, banana, ice cream, peanut butter, and malted milk powder in a blender, and mix on low speed until the mixture is blended. Continue mixing, gradually increasing the speed, until the mixture is smooth. Pour into glasses and garnish by inserting two Chocolate-Dipped Marshmallows (page 179) upright in each smoothie, if desired.

| | | | |
|---|---|---|---|
| Calories | 619 | Calcium | 252 mg |
| Calories from fat | 276 | Iron | 2 mg |
| Total fat | 31 g | Potassium | 1048 mg |
| Carbohydrates | 77 g | Magnesium | 131 mg |
| Protein | 17 g | Vitamin A | 170 mcg |
| Fiber | 5 g | Folic Acid | 68 mcg |

# Cappuccino Smoothie

*Surprise your guests with a Cappuccino Smoothie served in a deliciously edible Chocolate Bag (page 174).*

**2 SERVINGS**

3 tablespoons espresso or double-strength coffee, well chilled

2 tablespoons lowfat milk

1 cup sliced banana (1 large banana)

2 cups coffee ice cream

Place the coffee, milk, and banana in a blender, and mix on low speed until the banana is pureed. Add the ice cream and continue to mix, gradually increasing the speed, just until the mixture is blended. Place a Chocolate Bag (or champagne flute) on a small dessert plate and carefully divide the smoothie between the two Chocolate Bags (or flutes). Garnish each plate with a Strawberry Fan (page 212) or a White Chocolate–Dipped Strawberry (page 213), if desired.

| | | | |
|---|---|---|---|
| Calories | 616 | Calcium | 233 mg |
| Calories from fat | 311 | Iron | 1 mg |
| Total fat | 35 g | Potassium | 713 mg |
| Carbohydrates | 64 g | Magnesium | 23 mg |
| Protein | 11 g | Vitamin A | 227 mcg |
| Fiber | 2 g | Folic Acid | 14 mcg |

# Chocolate and Banana Monkey Tail

*Who doesn't love a chocolate-covered banana on a stick? Now it's even better made into a delicious smoothie.*

2 SERVINGS

6 tablespoons lowfat milk

1 tablespoon honey

1 ¼ teaspoons vanilla extract

3 cups sliced banana (3 large bananas)

1 cup vanilla lowfat frozen yogurt

1 cup chocolate lowfat frozen yogurt*

Place the milk, honey, vanilla, banana, and vanilla yogurt in a blender, and mix on low speed until the mixture is blended. Continue mixing, gradually increasing the speed, until the mixture is smooth.

Place the chocolate yogurt (or syrup) in a medium mixing bowl, and beat with a handheld electric beater until smooth.

| | | | |
|---|---|---|---|
| Calories | 483 | Calcium | 368 mg |
| Calories from fat | 47 | Iron | 2 mg |
| Total fat | 5 g | Potassium | 1485 mg |
| Carbohydrates | 103 g | Beta Carotene | 108 mcg |
| Protein | 13 g | Magnesium | 118 mg |
| Fiber | 7 g | Folic Acid | 63 mcg |

Pour half of the smoothie into cocktail glasses, then spoon the chocolate yogurt over each. Pour the remaining smoothie over the chocolate yogurt. Garnish each by inserting a Chocolate-Dipped Tortilla Triangle (page 181) upright in the smoothie, if desired.

*Chocolate syrup can be substituted for the chocolate yogurt. Follow the same steps, but spoon a tablespoon or more of the chocolate syrup between the layers of the smoothie. The smoothie can also be poured into a glass with chocolate syrup swirled over the top.

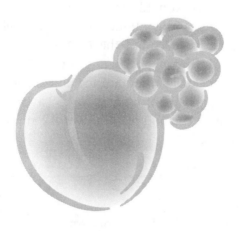

# Chocolate Peanut Butter Cup Smoothie

*Who can resist a chocolate peanut butter cup? Tiny chunks of these delicious morsels are blended into a rich filling of banana smoothie for the ultimate in decadence!*

### 2 SERVINGS

¼ cup lowfat milk

1 tablespoon honey

1 cup sliced banana (1 large banana)

2 cups vanilla ice cream

2 packages (1.6 ounces each) chocolate peanut butter cups, crushed

Place the milk, honey, and banana in a blender, and mix on low speed until the banana is pureed. Add the ice cream and continue to mix, gradually increasing the speed, until the mixture is smooth. Add the peanut butter cups; mix just until blended. Pour into cocktail glasses. For the ultimate in decadence, cut a narrow wedge out of a chocolate peanut butter cup and place it over the rim of the glass, if desired.

| | | | |
|---|---|---|---|
| Calories | 653 | Calcium | 247 mg |
| Calories from fat | 280 | Iron | 1 mg |
| Total fat | 31 g | Potassium | 792 mg |
| Carbohydrates | 86 g | Magnesium | 85 mg |
| Protein | 12 g | Vitamin A | 189 mcg |
| Fiber | 3 g | Folic Acid | 49 mcg |

# Copa-Banana Smoothie

*Sit back, enjoy the show, and let this smoothie entertain you.*

## 2 SERVINGS

¼ cup lowfat milk

1½ tablespoons chocolate syrup

1 cup sliced banana (1 large banana)

2 cups chocolate lowfat yogurt

2 tablespoons chocolate malted milk powder

½ teaspoon cinnamon

Place the milk, chocolate syrup, banana, yogurt, malted milk powder, and cinnamon in a blender, and mix on low speed until the mixture is blended. Continue mixing, gradually increasing the speed, until the mixture is smooth. Pour into glasses and garnish each by inserting a shard of chocolate lace* upright in the smoothie, if desired.

*Chocolate lace is a crispy, lacy pattern of caramelized sugar that is covered with a chocolate glaze. It is available in most fine candy stores.

| | | | |
|---|---|---|---|
| Calories | 412 | Calcium | 145 mg |
| Calories from fat | 39 | Iron | 0.81 mg |
| Total fat | 4 g | Potassium | 510 mg |
| Carbohydrates | 90 g | Beta Carotene | 37 mcg |
| Protein | 12 g | Magnesium | 42 mg |
| Fiber | 4 g | Vitamin A | 43 mcg |

# Creamy Caramel and Mocha Pleasure

*Your favorite coffeehouse mocha-caramel latte is even better as a smoothie.*

2 SERVINGS

½ cup lowfat milk

2 tablespoons coffee syrup

1 tablespoon honey

1 cup sliced banana (1 large banana)

2 cups vanilla ice cream

½ cup caramel topping

Place the milk, coffee syrup, honey, banana, ice cream, and caramel topping in a blender, and mix on low speed until the mixture is blended. Continue mixing, gradually increasing the speed, until the mixture is smooth. Pour into glasses and garnish each by inserting an Espresso Brittle Shard (page 193) upright in the smoothie, if desired.

| | | | |
|---|---|---|---|
| Calories | 643 | Calcium | 287 mg |
| Calories from fat | 146 | Iron | 0.84 mg |
| Total fat | 16 g | Potassium | 749 mg |
| Carbohydrates | 124 g | Beta Carotene | 36 mcg |
| Protein | 9 g | Magnesium | 47 mg |
| Fiber | 3 g | Vitamin A | 220 mcg |

# Fudge and Peanut Butter Blizzard

*You won't be stranded by this blizzard, but be prepared to be knocked off your feet by the delightful combinations of flavors.*

## 2 SERVINGS

½ cup lowfat milk

¼ cup chocolate syrup

1 cup sliced banana (1 large banana)

⅓ cup reduced-fat peanut butter

1 ½ cups vanilla fat-free frozen yogurt

Place the milk, chocolate syrup, banana, and peanut butter in a blender, and mix on low speed until the banana is pureed. Add the yogurt and continue to mix, gradually increasing the speed, until the mixture is smooth. Pour into glasses and garnish by inserting two Chocolate-Dipped Marshmallows (page 179) upright in each smoothie, if desired.

| | | | | |
|---|---|---|---|---|
| Calories | 563 | Calcium | 346 mg |
| Calories from fat | 149 | Iron | 2 mg |
| Total fat | 17 g | Potassium | 1027 mg |
| Carbohydrates | 87 g | Beta Carotene | 36 mcg |
| Protein | 23 g | Magnesium | 46 mg |
| Fiber | 5 g | Vitamin A | 46 mcg |

# Halvah-Nagila Smoothie

*Halvah is a Middle Eastern sweet made of sesame seeds and honey, found in most delicatessens or Asian or Middle Eastern food shops. After one taste of this exotic treat, you'll want to dance in a circle and sing its praises.*

### 2 SERVINGS

½ cup lowfat milk

1 cup sliced banana (1 large banana)

½ cup halvah, broken into small pieces

2 cups Starbucks Cashew Crunch ice cream, or other vanilla ice cream

Place the milk, banana, and halvah in a blender, and mix on low speed until the banana and halvah are pureed. Add the ice cream and continue to mix, gradually increasing the speed, until the mixture is smooth. Pour into glasses and garnish by inserting two Cinnamon-Coated Fusilli (page 187) upright in each smoothie, if desired.

| | | | |
|---|---|---|---|
| Calories | 927 | Calcium | 290 mg |
| Calories from fat | 412 | Iron | 4 mg |
| Total fat | 46 g | Potassium | 506 mg |
| Carbohydrates | 115 g | Magnesium | 145 mg |
| Protein | 20 g | Vitamin A | 1544 mcg |
| Fiber | 4 g | Folic Acid | 51 mcg |

# Heath Bar Hummer

*Anything made with crushed Heath bars has to be the ultimate delight.*

### 2 SERVINGS

1 cup sliced banana (1 large banana)

2 cups Starbucks Dulce de Leche ice cream, or other caramel ice cream

2 packages (1.4 ounces each) Heath bars, or other chocolate-covered toffee candy bars, crushed

Place the banana in a blender, and mix on low speed until pureed. Add the ice cream and continue to mix, gradually increasing the speed, until the mixture is smooth. Add the Heath bars; mix just to blend. Pour into glasses and garnish each by inserting a Chocolate Heart (page 183) upright in the smoothie, if desired.

| Calories | 861 | Calcium | 305 mg |
| Calories from fat | 428 | Iron | 0.23 mg |
| Total fat | 48 g | Potassium | 297 mg |
| Carbohydrates | 97 g | Beta Carotene | 36 mcg |
| Protein | 13 g | Magnesium | 22 mg |
| Fiber | 2 g | Vitamin A | 1006 mcg |

# I Am the Walnut

*We're all together when we agree this is one of the best smoothies ever tasted.*

2 SERVINGS

¼ cup walnuts

¼ cup lowfat milk

3 tablespoons chocolate syrup

1 cup sliced banana (1 large banana)

2 cups vanilla ice cream

Place the walnuts in the blender and finely chop. Add the milk, chocolate syrup, and banana, and mix on medium speed until the banana is pureed. Add the ice cream and continue to mix, gradually increasing the speed, until the mixture is smooth. Pour into glasses and garnish each by inserting a Chocolate-Dipped Tortilla Triangle (page 181) upright in the smoothie, if desired.

| | | | |
|---|---|---|---|
| Calories | 522 | Calcium | 221 mg |
| Calories from fat | 222 | Iron | 1 mg |
| Total fat | 25 g | Potassium | 693 mg |
| Carbohydrates | 70 g | Beta Carotene | 64 mcg |
| Protein | 11 g | Magnesium | 72 mg |
| Fiber | 3 g | Vitamin A | 184 mcg |

# Lady Banana

*You don't have to be a Beatles fan to enjoy this heavenly delight (but it doesn't hurt). It can be served in a glass or, to make it more exciting, in a Chocolate Bag (page 174) garnished with a Pirouette cookie (page 209).*

### 2 SERVINGS

¾ cup lowfat milk

1 tablespoon honey

2 cups sliced banana (2 large bananas)

1 cup vanilla lowfat frozen yogurt

1 tablespoon chocolate malted milk powder

Place the milk, honey, banana, yogurt, and malted milk powder in a blender, and mix on low speed until the mixture is blended. Continue mixing, gradually increasing the speed, until the mixture is smooth. Pour into wine goblets (or a Chocolate Bag) and garnish each with a Chocolate-Covered Spoon (page 176), if desired.

| | | | |
|---|---|---|---|
| Calories | 360 | Calcium | 271 mg |
| Calories from fat | 39 | Iron | 0.82 mg |
| Total fat | 4 g | Potassium | 1015 mg |
| Carbohydrates | 76 g | Beta Carotene | 72 mcg |
| Protein | 10 g | Magnesium | 66 mg |
| Fiber | 4 g | Vitamin A | 84 mcg |

# Livin' La Vida Mocha

*You'll want your dancing shoes after indulging in this seductively delicious smoothie.*

2 SERVINGS

½ cup lowfat milk

1 tablespoon coffee syrup

1 tablespoon chocolate syrup

½ teaspoon vanilla extract

1 cup sliced banana (1 large banana)

2 cups coffee ice cream

Place the milk, coffee syrup, chocolate syrup, vanilla, and banana in a blender, and mix on low speed until the banana is pureed. Add the ice cream and continue to mix, gradually increasing the speed, until the mixture is smooth. Pour into wine goblets and garnish each by inserting an Espresso Brittle Shard (page 192) upright in the smoothie.

| | | | | |
|---|---|---|---|---|
| Calories | 687 | Calcium | 287 mg |
| Calories from fat | 320 | Iron | 1 mg |
| Total fat | 36 g | Potassium | 786 mg |
| Carbohydrates | 77 g | Beta Carotene | 36 mcg |
| Protein | 13 g | Vitamin A | 256 mcg |
| Fiber | 2 g | Vitamin D IU | 25 IU |

# Oreo Cookie Monster Smoothie

*Don't be a grouch and eat all the cookies before they are mixed into this marvelous indulgence.*

### 2 SERVINGS

¼ cup lowfat milk

1 ½ cups vanilla fat-free frozen yogurt

1 cup sliced banana (1 large banana)

10 Oreo cookies, crumbled

Place the milk, yogurt, and banana in a blender, and mix on low speed until just blended. Add the cookies and mix just to blend. Pour into cocktail glasses and garnish each by inserting an Oreo cookie upright in the smoothie, if desired.

| | | | |
|---|---|---|---|
| Calories | 495 | Calcium | 289 mg |
| Calories from fat | 116 | Iron | 2 mg |
| Total fat | 13 g | Potassium | 770 mg |
| Carbohydrates | 86 g | Beta Carotene | 36 mcg |
| Protein | 12 g | Magnesium | 46 mg |
| Fiber | 3 g | Folic Acid | 30 mcg |

# Peanut Butter Decadence

*The name of this smoothie says it all. Lots of peanut butter mixed with ice cream cannot be topped.*

2 SERVINGS

¾ cup lowfat milk

1 tablespoon honey

1 ½ cups sliced banana (2 large bananas)

1 cup chocolate or vanilla ice cream

½ cup creamy peanut butter

Place the milk, honey, banana, ice cream, and peanut butter in a blender, and mix on low speed until the mixture is blended. Continue mixing, gradually increasing the speed, until the mixture is smooth. Pour into wine goblets and garnish by inserting a Chocolate-Dipped Tortilla Triangle (page 181) upright in the smoothie, if desired.

| | | | |
|---|---|---|---|
| Calories | 707 | Calcium | 205 mg |
| Calories from fat | 381 | Iron | 2 mg |
| Total fat | 42 g | Potassium | 1197 mg |
| Carbohydrates | 71 g | Magnesium | 154 mg |
| Protein | 23 g | Vitamin A | 144 mcg |
| Fiber | 7 g | Folic Acid | 80 mcg |

# The Pear Essentials

*This is all you need to satisfy a craving for a sweet indulgence.*

2 SERVINGS

### Sautéed Pears

1 tablespoon butter

2 cups peeled and diced pear (2 large pears)

2 tablespoons granulated sugar

2 tablespoons firmly packed brown sugar

⅛ teaspoon cinnamon

1 tablespoon apple liqueur

### Smoothie

½ cup lowfat milk

Sautéed pears

½ teaspoon vanilla extract

¼ teaspoon cinnamon

1½ cups vanilla fat-free frozen yogurt

| | | | |
|---|---|---|---|
| Calories | 453 | Calcium | 355 mg |
| Calories from fat | 71 | Iron | 1 mg |
| Total fat | 8 g | Potassium | 685 mg |
| Carbohydrates | 86 g | Vitamin A | 97 mcg |
| Protein | 10 g | Vitamin D | 28 IU |
| Fiber | 4 g | Folic Acid | 28 mcg |

**To make sautéed pears**
Melt butter in an 8-inch sauté pan over medium heat. Increase heat to high and add pears, sugars, and cinnamon; sauté for 5 to 6 minutes or until pears begin to caramelize, stirring frequently. Add the apple liqueur and cook for 1 minute. Remove the pan from heat and allow the pears to come to room temperature. When cool, transfer the pears and sauce to a plastic wrap–lined plate and freeze for 1 hour.

**To make the smoothie**
Place the milk, sautéed pears, vanilla, and cinnamon in a blender, and mix on low speed until the pears are pureed. Add the yogurt and continue to mix, gradually increasing the speed, until the mixture is smooth. Pour into cocktail glasses and garnish by inserting two Cinnamon-Coated Fusilli upright in each smoothie, if desired (page 187).

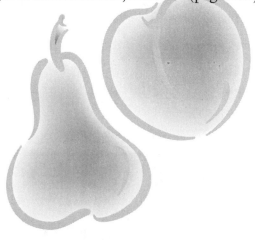

# Turtle Tornado

*Gooey caramel and luscious pecans coated with chocolate are the ultimate candy treat. Combining these same ingredients in a smoothie is just as sensational.*

## 2 SERVINGS

3 tablespoons pecans

½ cup lowfat milk

2 cups chocolate ice cream

5 tablespoons caramel topping

Place the pecans in a blender and finely chop. Add the milk, ice cream, and caramel topping, and mix on medium speed until the mixture is smooth. Pour into wine goblets and garnish each by inserting a chocolate lace shard* upright in the smoothie, if desired.

*Chocolate lace is a crispy, lacy pattern of caramelized sugar that is covered with a chocolate glaze. It is available in most fine candy stores.

| | | | |
|---|---|---|---|
| Calories | 521 | Calcium | 243 mg |
| Calories from fat | 210 | Iron | 2 mg |
| Total fat | 23 g | Potassium | 518 mg |
| Carbohydrates | 76 g | Magnesium | 56 mg |
| Protein | 9 g | Vitamin A | 210 mcg |
| Fiber | 3 g | Vitamin D | 46 IU |

# CHAPTER 8

# Black Tie Only

## Smoothies Go Uptown

*T*he idea of serving a smoothie at a formal event may sound like the ultimate oxymoron, but when a hint of liqueur is blended with traditional smoothie ingredients, the drink can achieve a new dimension in taste and distinction. Not only does the smoothie acquire a refreshingly unique taste, but imagine the elegance when your creation is served in a Chocolate Bag, garnished with a Chocolate Heart, or placed on a dessert plate with a White Chocolate–Dipped Strawberry set beside the glass.

In this chapter, you will be enticed by over twenty recipes for company-quality smoothies such as Irish Coffee Jig, Amaretto Peach Passion, and Won't You Come Home Banana Bailey. Unlike Agent 007, your guests will be both shaken and stirred by these surprisingly exotic creations with a little bite.

# Amaretto Peach Passion

*This special smoothie is thick enough to serve in a Chocolate Bag (page 174); however, a pretty glass also works well.*

### 2 SERVINGS

½ cup lowfat milk

3 tablespoons amaretto, or other almond liqueur

1 tablespoon honey

1 teaspoon vanilla extract

2 cups peeled and diced peach (2 large peaches)

2 cups peach lowfat frozen yogurt

Place the milk, almond liqueur, honey, vanilla, and peach in a blender, and mix on low speed until the peaches are pureed. Add the yogurt and continue to mix, gradually increasing the speed, until the mixture is smooth. Spoon into Chocolate Bags or champagne flutes and garnish by inserting two reception sticks* upright in each smoothie, if desired.

| | | | |
|---|---|---|---|
| Calories | 423 | Calcium | 384 mg |
| Calories from fat | 37 | Iron | 0.40 mg |
| Total fat | 4 g | Potassium | 842 mg |
| Carbohydrates | 77 g | Beta Carotene | 452 mcg |
| Protein | 12 g | Magnesium | 42 mg |
| Fiber | 3 g | Vitamin A | 156 mcg |

*Reception sticks are chocolate-dipped crisp candy sticks that come in a variety of flavors, such as mint, orange, cinnamon, and lemon. They are available in most fine candy shops.

# Banana Banshee

*This smoothie is quick and easy to prepare and, at the same time, delicious and elegant.*

### 2 SERVINGS

½ cup crème de cacao

2 cups sliced banana (2 large bananas)

1 ½ cups vanilla ice cream

Place the crème de cacao and banana in a blender, and mix on low speed until the banana is pureed. Add the ice cream and continue to mix, gradually increasing the speed, until the mixture is smooth. Pour into champagne flutes and garnish each by inserting a Pirouette cookie (page 209) upright in the smoothie, if desired.

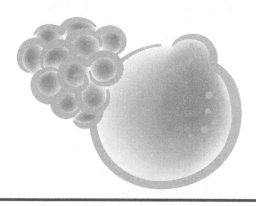

| Calories | 537 | Calcium | 136 mg |
|---|---|---|---|
| Calories from fat | 106 | Iron | 0.59 mg |
| Total fat | 12 g | Potassium | 800 mg |
| Carbohydrates | 84 g | Beta Carotene | 72 mcg |
| Protein | 5 g | Magnesium | 58 mg |
| Fiber | 4 g | Vitamin A | 128 mcg |

# Banana Daiquiri

*Impress your friends by serving them this delicious smoothie before or after dinner.*

2 SERVINGS

½ cup lowfat milk

3 to 4 tablespoons dark rum

2 cups sliced banana (2 large bananas)

2 cups banana lowfat frozen yogurt

Place the milk, rum, and banana in a blender, and mix on low speed until the banana is pureed. Add the yogurt and continue to mix, gradually increasing the speed, until the mixture is smooth. Pour into cocktail glasses and garnish by inserting two Cinnamon-Coated Fusilli (page 187) upright in each smoothie, if desired.

| | | | |
|---|---|---|---|
| Calories | 422 | Calcium | 383 mg |
| Calories from fat | 41 | Iron | 0.64 mg |
| Total fat | 5 g | Potassium | 1090 mg |
| Carbohydrates | 75 g | Beta Carotene | 72 mcg |
| Protein | 12 g | Magnesium | 73 mg |
| Fiber | 4 g | Vitamin A | 76 mcg |

# Banana Rum-Ba

*Put on your dancing shoes, because after you have tasted this heavenly delight, your feet will start involuntarily tapping.*

### 2 SERVINGS

¼ cup lowfat milk

2 tablespoons light rum

2 tablespoons white crème de cacao

2 tablespoons crème de banana, or other banana liqueur

2 cups sliced banana (2 large bananas)

1½ cups vanilla fat-free frozen yogurt

Place the milk, rum, crème de cacao, banana liqueur, and banana in a blender, and mix on low speed until the banana is pureed. Add the yogurt and continue to mix, gradually increasing the speed, until the mixture is smooth. Pour into cocktail glasses and garnish each by inserting a Chocolate-Dipped Tortilla Triangle (page 181) upright in the smoothie, if desired.

| | | | | |
|---|---|---|---|---|
| Calories | 430 | Calcium | 294 mg |
| Calories from fat | 15 | Iron | 0.62 mg |
| Total fat | 2 g | Potassium | 971 mg |
| Carbohydrates | 78 g | Beta Carotene | 72 mcg |
| Protein | 10 g | Magnesium | 68 mg |
| Fiber | 4 g | Folic Acid | 44 mcg |

# Banana and Strawberry Seduction

*This seductively easy-to-prepare smoothie will be hard to resist.*

2 SERVINGS

6 tablespoons crème de banana, or other banana liqueur

1 cup sliced banana (1 large banana)

1 cup diced strawberries

2 cups vanilla fat-free frozen yogurt

Place the banana liqueur, banana, strawberries, and yogurt in a blender, and mix on low speed until the mixture is blended. Continue mixing, gradually increasing the speed, until the mixture is smooth. Pour into champagne flutes and garnish the rim of each glass with a Strawberry Fan (page 212), if desired.

| | | | |
|---|---|---|---|
| Calories | 435 | Calcium | 351 mg |
| Calories from fat | 10 | Iron | 0.74 mg |
| Total fat | 1 g | Potassium | 870 mg |
| Carbohydrates | 80 g | Beta Carotene | 49 mcg |
| Protein | 11 g | Magnesium | 63 mg |
| Fiber | 4 g | Vitamin C | 55 mg |

# Bananas Foster

*A special smoothie to serve when you want to impress your guests with a dessert that is richly delicious and elegant.*

2 SERVINGS

½ cup lowfat milk

1 tablespoon dark rum

½ tablespoon crème de banana, or other banana liqueur

½ tablespoon honey

2 cups sliced banana (2 large bananas)

1 tablespoon dark brown sugar

⅛ teaspoon cinnamon

1 cup banana lowfat frozen yogurt

Place the milk, rum, banana liqueur, honey, banana, brown sugar, and cinnamon in a blender, and mix on low speed until the banana is pureed. Add the yogurt and continue to mix, gradually increasing the speed, until the mixture is smooth. Pour into brandy balloon glasses and garnish each with a Cinnamon Wonton Crisp (page 189), if desired.

| | | | |
|---|---|---|---|
| Calories | 343 | Calcium | 238 mg |
| Calories from fat | 30 | Iron | 0.76 mg |
| Total fat | 3 g | Potassium | 921 mg |
| Carbohydrates | 70 g | Beta Carotene | 72 mcg |
| Protein | 8 g | Magnesium | 60 mg |
| Fiber | 4 g | Vitamin A | 63 mcg |

# Bedazzling Raspberry Smoothie

*Dazzle your guests with this sophisticated smoothie.*

2 SERVINGS

¾ cup lowfat milk

1 tablespoon Chambord, or other raspberry liqueur

2 cups raspberries

2 tablespoons raspberry preserves

1½ cups vanilla fat-free frozen yogurt

Place the milk, raspberry liqueur, raspberries, and raspberry preserves in a blender, and mix on low speed until the raspberries are pureed. Add the yogurt and continue to mix, gradually increasing the speed, until the mixture is smooth. Pour into champagne flutes and garnish each by inserting a Pirouette cookie (page 209) upright in the smoothie, if desired.

| | | | |
|---|---|---|---|
| Calories | 327 | Calcium | 379 mg |
| Calories from fat | 25 | Iron | 0.83 mg |
| Total fat | 3 g | Potassium | 683 mg |
| Carbohydrates | 64 g | Beta Carotene | 48 mcg |
| Protein | 11 g | Vitamin A | 75 mcg |
| Fiber | 8 g | Folic Acid | 47 mcg |

# Blackberry Tie Only

*When your invitation requests formal attire for a special event, this well-appointed smoothie can rise to the occasion. It is delicious served in a Chocolate Bag (page 174) or just as divine in a pretty glass.*

2 SERVINGS

¼ cup crème de cassis

2 tablespoons honey

2 cups blackberries

2 cups vanilla fat-free frozen yogurt

Place the crème de cassis, honey, and blackberries in a blender, and mix on low speed until the blackberries are pureed. Add the yogurt and continue to mix, gradually increasing the speed, just until the mixture is smooth. Pour into champagne flutes and garnish by inserting two Cinnamon-Coated Fusilli (page 187) upright in each smoothie, if desired.

| | | | |
|---|---|---|---|
| Calories | 435 | Calcium | 382 mg |
| Calories from fat | 9 | Iron | 1 mg |
| Total fat | 0.95 g | Potassium | 722 mg |
| Carbohydrates | 86 g | Beta Carotene | 69 mcg |
| Protein | 11 g | Vitamin C | 32 mg |
| Fiber | 8 g | Folic Acid | 70 mcg |

# Brandy Alexander

*You will adore this sophisticated smoothie made with the same ingredients as those found in the popular Brandy Alexander cocktail.*

2 SERVINGS

¼ cup coffee syrup

2 tablespoons brandy

2 tablespoons crème de cacao

1 cup sliced banana (1 large banana)

2 cups vanilla or chocolate lowfat frozen yogurt

Place the coffee syrup, brandy, crème de cacao, and banana in a blender, and mix on low speed until the banana is pureed. Add the yogurt and continue to mix, gradually increasing the speed, until the mixture is smooth. Pour into brandy balloon glasses and garnish each by inserting a Marbleized Chocolate Shard (page 200) upright in the smoothie, if desired.

| | | | |
|---|---|---|---|
| Calories | 429 | Calcium | 316 mg |
| Calories from fat | 27 | Iron | 0.96 mg |
| Total fat | 3 g | Potassium | 718 mg |
| Carbohydrates | 79 g | Beta Carotene | 36 mcg |
| Protein | 10 g | Magnesium | 53 mg |
| Fiber | 2 g | Folic Acid | 33 mcg |

# Caramel Miranda Apple Smoothie

*This smoothie is the next best thing to a caramel apple on a stick. It is worth the extra effort to caramelize the apples before adding them to the smoothie. Best of all, when you're done enjoying this delicious throwback to your childhood, your mother won't have to wipe your face.*

2 SERVINGS

### Caramelized Apples

1½ tablespoons unsalted butter

3 cups peeled and diced Granny Smith apple
  (3 large apples)

6 tablespoons granulated sugar

3 tablespoons Calvados, or other apple liqueur

### Smoothie

¼ cup lowfat milk

Caramelized apples

1½ cups vanilla fat-free frozen yogurt

¼ teaspoon nutmeg

¼ teaspoon cinnamon

⅛ teaspoon allspice

| | | | |
|---|---|---|---|
| Calories | 530 | Calcium | 301 mg |
| Calories from fat | 87 | Iron | 0.63 mg |
| Total fat | 10 g | Potassium | 562 mg |
| Carbohydrates | 98 g | Magnesium | 32 mg |
| Protein | 9 g | Vitamin A | 103 mcg |
| Fiber | 3 g | Vitamin D | 18 IU |

**To make the caramelized apples**
Melt the butter in a medium nonstick pan over medium-high heat. Add the apples and sugar and sauté for 5 to 7 minutes or until the mixture begins to caramelize, stirring frequently. Add the apple liqueur and boil for 40 seconds. Allow the apples to cool in the pan. Transfer the apples to a plate lined with plastic wrap and place in the freezer for 1 hour.

**To make the smoothie**
Place the milk, caramelized apples, yogurt, nutmeg, cinnamon, and allspice in a blender, and mix on low speed until the mixture is blended. Continue to mix, gradually increasing the speed, until the mixture is smooth. Pour into champagne flutes and garnish each by inserting a 6-inch cinnamon stick upright in the smoothie, if desired.

# Cherries Jubilee

*Cherries Jubilee has been a favorite dessert for a long time. Using the same ingredients in a smoothie can make it an excellent dessert to serve after a filling meal.*

2 SERVINGS

¾ cup white grape juice

1 tablespoon honey

2 cups stemmed and seeded Bing cherries

2 cups vanilla fat-free frozen yogurt

½ teaspoon vanilla extract

Place the juice, honey, cherries, yogurt, and vanilla in a blender, and mix on low speed until the mixture is blended. Continue mixing, gradually increasing the speed, until the mixture is smooth. Pour into cocktail glasses and garnish each by inserting a Pirouette cookie (page 209) upright in the smoothie, if desired.

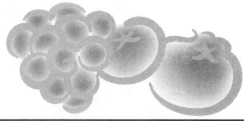

| Calories | 388 | Calcium | 366 mg |
|---|---|---|---|
| Calories from fat | 16 | Iron | 1 mg |
| Total fat | 1.77 g | Potassium | 886 mg |
| Carbohydrates | 85 g | Beta Carotene | 174 mcg |
| Protein | 12 g | Magnesium | 58 mg |
| Fiber | 3 g | Vitamin A | 35 mcg |

# Chocolate Black Russian

*Calorie-free?* Nyet. *Delicious and elegant?* Da!

**2** SERVINGS

2 tablespoons Kahlúa, or other coffee liqueur

2 tablespoons vodka

1 cup sliced banana (1 large banana)

1¾ cups chocolate ice cream

Place the coffee liqueur, vodka, and banana in a blender, and mix on low speed until the banana is pureed. Add the ice cream and continue to mix, gradually increasing the speed, until the mixture is smooth. Pour into champagne flutes and garnish each by inserting a Chocolate Heart (page 183) upright in the smoothie, if desired.

| | | | |
|---|---|---|---|
| Calories | 401 | Calcium | 130 mg |
| Calories from fat | 118 | Iron | 1 mg |
| Total fat | 13 g | Potassium | 587 mg |
| Carbohydrates | 56 g | Beta Carotene | 36 mcg |
| Protein | 5 g | Magnesium | 55 mg |
| Fiber | 3 g | Vitamin A | 143 mcg |

# Cloud Nine

*Is this heaven? No, but this celestial smoothie comes pretty close.*

2 SERVINGS

2 tablespoons Baileys Original Irish Cream, or other Irish cream liqueur

1 tablespoon Chambord, or other raspberry liqueur

1 tablespoon amaretto, or other almond liqueur

1 cup sliced banana (1 large banana)

2 cups vanilla ice cream

Place the Irish cream liqueur, raspberry liqueur, almond liqueur, and banana in a blender, and mix on low speed until the banana is pureed. Add the ice cream and continue to mix, gradually increasing the speed, until the mixture is smooth. Pour into cocktail glasses and garnish each by inserting an Espresso Brittle Shard (page 193) upright in the smoothie, if desired.

| | | | | |
|---|---|---|---|---|
| Calories | 423 | Calcium | 191 mg |
| Calories from fat | 157 | Iron | 0.40 mg |
| Total fat | 17 g | Potassium | 562 mg |
| Carbohydrates | 58 g | Beta Carotene | 36 mcg |
| Protein | 6 g | Magnesium | 40 mg |
| Fiber | 2 g | Vitamin A | 176 mcg |

# Grand Marnier Razzamatazz

*Raspberries and Grand Marnier team up to make an exquisite smoothie.*

2 SERVINGS

½ cup orange juice

3 tablespoons Grand Marnier, or other orange-flavored liqueur

2 tablespoons honey

2 cups raspberries

2 cups Häagen-Dazs Vanilla Raspberry Swirl fat-free frozen yogurt, or other vanilla raspberry frozen yogurt

Place the juice, orange liqueur, honey, raspberries, and yogurt in a blender, and mix on low speed until the mixture is blended. Continue mixing, gradually increasing the speed, until the mixture is smooth. Pour into champagne flutes and garnish each by inserting a Pirouette cookie (page 209) upright in the smoothie, if desired.

| | | | |
|---|---|---|---|
| Calories | 488 | Calcium | 235 mg |
| Calories from fat | 8 | Iron | 0.93 mg |
| Total fat | 0.86 g | Potassium | 325 mg |
| Carbohydrates | 104 g | Beta Carotene | 71 mcg |
| Protein | 10 g | Vitamin C | 62 mg |
| Fiber | 9 g | Folic Acid | 51 mcg |

# Irish-Banana-Man Chill

*As chilled as this smoothie may be, it will make you feel warm and satisfied inside.*

2 SERVINGS

¼ cup coffee syrup

2 tablespoons Baileys Original Irish Cream, or other Irish cream liqueur

1 tablespoon Irish whiskey

1 cup sliced banana (1 large banana)

2 cups vanilla lowfat frozen yogurt

Place the coffee syrup, Irish cream liqueur, Irish whiskey, and banana in a blender, and mix on low speed until the banana is pureed. Add the yogurt and continue to mix, gradually increasing the speed, until the mixture is smooth. Pour into champagne flutes or wine goblets and garnish each by inserting a Chocolate-Dipped Tortilla Triangle (page 181) upright in the smoothie, if desired.

| | | | |
|---|---|---|---|
| Calories | 401 | Calcium | 333 mg |
| Calories from fat | 49 | Iron | 0.99 mg |
| Total fat | 5 g | Potassium | 716 mg |
| Carbohydrates | 76 g | Beta Carotene | 36 mcg |
| Protein | 10 g | Magnesium | 53 mg |
| Fiber | 2 g | Vitamin A | 48 mcg |

# *Irish Coffee Jig*

*A spirited river dance will come to mind after one taste of this richly coffee-flavored smoothie with a delicious hint of Irish whiskey. If you really like whiskey, add slightly more than the recommended amount.*

2 SERVINGS

¼ cup Irish whiskey

2 tablespoons lowfat milk

I cup sliced banana (I large banana)

2 cups coffee ice cream

Place the Irish whiskey, milk, and banana in a blender, and mix on medium speed until the banana is pureed. Add the ice cream and mix just until blended. Pour into glasses and garnish each by inserting an Espresso Brittle Shard (page 193) upright in the smoothie, if desired.

| | | | |
|---|---|---|---|
| Calories | 681 | Calcium | 233 mg |
| Calories from fat | 311 | Iron | I mg |
| Total fat | 35 g | Potassium | 702 mg |
| Carbohydrates | 64 g | Beta Carotene | 36 mcg |
| Protein | II g | Magnesium | 22 mg |
| Fiber | 2 g | Vitamin A | 227 mcg |

# Mocha Coffee Delight

*This delicious smoothie can be the crowning touch to a memorable evening.*

### 2 SERVINGS

¼ cup hot water

2 tablespoons instant coffee granules

1½ cups lowfat milk

2 tablespoons chocolate syrup

1 tablespoon honey

1 cup sliced banana (1 large banana)

2 cups vanilla fat-free frozen yogurt

Coffee liqueur, to taste (optional)

Combine the water and coffee granules and blend well. Set aside to cool to room temperature.

Place the milk, dissolved coffee, chocolate syrup, honey, and banana in a blender, and mix on low speed until the banana is pureed. Add the yogurt and optional coffee liqueur, and continue to mix, gradually increasing the speed, until the

| | | | |
|---|---|---|---|
| Calories | 454 | Calcium | 553 mg |
| Calories from fat | 42 | Iron | 0.97 mg |
| Total fat | 5 g | Potassium | 1229 mg |
| Carbohydrates | 88 g | Magnesium | 72 mg |
| Protein | 18 g | Vitamin A | 122 mcg |
| Fiber | 2 g | Vitamin D | 74 IU |

mixture is smooth. Pour into cocktail glasses and place each one on a dessert plate. Garnish each plate with a White Chocolate–Dipped Strawberry (page 213), if desired.

# Mudslide Madness

*One glance at the tempting ingredients in this decadent smoothie, and you will understand why you'll fall madly in love with it.*

### 2 SERVINGS

2 tablespoons Kahlúa, or other coffee liqueur

2 tablespoons Baileys Original Irish Cream or other Irish cream liqueur

2 tablespoons vodka

1 cup sliced banana (1 large banana)

1½ cups vanilla fat-free frozen yogurt

12 Oreo cookies, crushed

Place the coffee liqueur, Irish cream liqueur, vodka, and banana in a blender, and mix on low speed until the banana is pureed. Add the yogurt and continue to mix, gradually increasing the speed, until the mixture is smooth Add the cookies and mix just to blend. Pour into cocktail glasses and garnish each by inserting an Oreo cookie upright in the smoothie, if desired.

| | | | | |
|---|---|---|---|---|
| Calories | 653 | Calcium | 273 mg |
| Calories from fat | 154 | Iron | 2 mg |
| Total fat | 17 g | Potassium | 741 mg |
| Carbohydrates | 101 g | Beta Carotene | 36 mcg |
| Protein | 13 g | Magnesium | 46 mg |
| Fiber | 4 g | Folic Acid | 30 mcg |

# Pineapple Daiquiri

*The perfect smoothie to enjoy with friends as you gather around the grill and enjoy a spirited conversation.*

### 2 SERVINGS

3 tablespoons light rum

3 tablespoons dark rum

1 tablespoon honey

1 teaspoon vanilla extract

2 cups diced pineapple (1 pineapple)

½ teaspoon cinnamon

2 cups pineapple lowfat frozen yogurt

Place the rums, honey, vanilla, pineapple, and cinnamon in a blender, and mix on low speed until the pineapple is pureed. Add the yogurt and continue to mix, gradually increasing the speed, until the mixture is smooth. Pour into cocktail glasses and garnish each by inserting a Pineapple Chip (page 205) upright in the smoothie, if desired.

| | | | |
|---|---|---|---|
| Calories | 416 | Calcium | 326 mg |
| Calories from fat | 30 | Iron | 1 mg |
| Total fat | 3 g | Potassium | 581 mg |
| Carbohydrates | 66 g | Magnesium | 52 mg |
| Protein | 10 g | Vitamin A | 30 mcg |
| Fiber | 2 g | Folic Acid | 36 mcg |

# Strawberry Daiquiri

*Enjoy this smoothie before or after dinner—or on any occasion when a special treat is in order.*

2 SERVINGS

¼ cup light rum

2 teaspoons fresh lime juice

2 cups diced strawberries

2 cups vanilla ice cream

Place the rum, juice, strawberries, and ice cream in a blender, and mix on low speed until the mixture is blended. Continue mixing, gradually increasing the speed, until the mixture is smooth. Pour into cocktail glasses and garnish the rim of each glass with a Strawberry Fan (page 212), if desired.

| | | | |
|---|---|---|---|
| Calories | 381 | Calcium | 193 mg |
| Calories from fat | 136 | Iron | 0.78 mg |
| Total fat | 15 g | Potassium | 544 mg |
| Carbohydrates | 43 g | Vitamin A | 160 mcg |
| Protein | 6 g | Vitamin C | 96 mg |
| Fiber | 4 g | Folic Acid | 36 mcg |

# Tequila Tornado

*After one sip of this spirited smoothie, Dorothy and Toto would have instantly realized that they were not in Kansas anymore.*

2 SERVINGS

2 tablespoons tequila

2 tablespoons pineapple juice

1 tablespoon grenadine

2 cups diced pineapple (1 pineapple)

2 cups pineapple lowfat frozen yogurt

Place the tequila, juice, grenadine, and pineapple in a blender, and mix on low speed until the mixture is blended. Add the yogurt and continue to mix, gradually increasing the speed, until the mixture is smooth. Pour into champagne flutes and garnish each with a Pineapple, Orange, and Cherry Blossom (page 207), if desired.

| Calories | 347 | Calcium | 321 mg |
|---|---|---|---|
| Calories from fat | 30 | Iron | 0.79 mg |
| Total fat | 3 g | Potassium | 593 mg |
| Carbohydrates | 65 g | Magnesium | 53 mg |
| Protein | 9 g | Vitamin A | 30 mcg |
| Fiber | 2 g | Folic Acid | 39 mcg |

# Tropical Tuxedo

*This smoothie is elegant enough to serve after a formal dinner. It is especially attractive when served in a hollowed-out pineapple or coconut shell.*

2 SERVINGS

½ cup pineapple juice

1 teaspoon fresh lime juice

¼ cup light coconut milk

3 tablespoons light rum

1 tablespoon honey

¼ teaspoon vanilla extract

1 cup peeled and diced papaya (1 large papaya)

1 cup sliced banana (1 large banana)

1 cup vanilla lowfat frozen yogurt

Place the juices, coconut milk, rum, honey, vanilla, papaya, banana, and yogurt in a blender, and mix on low speed until the mixture is blended. Continue mixing, gradually increasing the speed, until the mixture is smooth. Pour into champagne flutes and garnish each by inserting a Pineapple Chip (page 205) in the smoothie, if desired.

| | | | |
|---|---|---|---|
| Calories | 333 | Calcium | 186 mg |
| Calories from fat | 30 | Iron | 0.75 mg |
| Total fat | 3 g | Potassium | 767 mg |
| Carbohydrates | 62 g | Beta Carotene | 73 mcg |
| Protein | 6.23 g | Vitamin C | 58 mg |
| Fiber | 3 g | Folic Acid | 65 mcg |

# Won't You Come Home Banana Bailey

*You won't ever have to ask this question once you have served this sensational delight. One suggestion: Make extra, because it's so good.*

2 SERVINGS

¼ cup lowfat milk

2 tablespoon Baileys Original Irish Cream or other Irish cream liqueur

¼ teaspoon vanilla extract

2 cups sliced banana (1 large banana)

1½ cups vanilla ice cream

Place the milk, Irish cream liqueur, vanilla, and banana in a blender, and mix on low speed until the banana is pureed. Add the ice cream and continue to mix, gradually increasing the speed, until the mixture is smooth. Pour into cocktail glasses and garnish each by inserting a Pirouette cookie (page 209) upright in the smoothie, if desired.

| | | | |
|---|---|---|---|
| Calories | 393 | Calcium | 187 mg |
| Calories from fat | 132 | Iron | 0.60 mg |
| Total fat | 15 g | Potassium | 843 mg |
| Carbohydrates | 63 g | Beta Carotene | 72 mcg |
| Protein | 7 g | Magnesium | 57 mg |
| Fiber | 4 g | Vitamin A | 162 mcg |

CHAPTER **9**

# Garnishes with a Flourish

A well-chosen garnish can play an important role when you want to create something special out of a simple combination of smoothie ingredients. For those special occasions when you want to elevate a smoothie to a memorable dessert, present it in an attractive champagne flute or a dazzling Chocolate Bag and garnished with a Chocolate-Dipped Tortilla Triangle, a Chocolate Heart, or a Chocolate-Dipped Marshmallow. Even a basic fruit smoothie can be adorned with a Fruit Skewer or a Lemon and Cranberry Twist. Better yet, all of these garnishes themselves are exceptionally delicious. Are you tempted yet?

In this chapter, you will find a host of novel ideas for creating a variety of garnishes. While they perfectly dress up a smoothie, many can be used for one of your other favorite desserts as well, such as a sundae, mousse, or a simple dish of ice cream. If you don't have time to garnish, then you might consider picking up some fun accessories at your neighborhood party store such as multicolored and uniquely shaped straws, cocktail umbrellas, brightly colored metallic sparklers, or colored stirrers.

To garnish or not to garnish—that will no longer be the question once you see how easy it is and how impressive the results can be.

# Apple Chips

*Apple chips are crunchy, paper-thin slices of apples. They are the perfect garnish to dress up any smoothie. Not only do they add a sophisticated elegance to smoothies or other desserts, but they are delicious as well. The chips are best when apples are thinly sliced with a mandoline or vegetable slicer; however, with a little patience, a sharp knife can be just as effective.*

### 16 TO 20 CHIPS

1 Granny Smith or Golden Delicious apple, unpeeled and uncored

2 cups cold water

2 tablespoons fresh lemon juice

2 cups cold water

2 cups granulated sugar

2 tablespoons fresh lemon juice

**To make the Apple Chips**
Preheat oven to 200 degrees F.

Thinly slice the apples into horizontal rings, about 1/16-inch thick. Place the apple rings in a bowl filled with 2 cups water and 2 tablespoons lemon juice. Set aside.

| | | | |
|---|---|---|---|
| Calories | 10 | Calcium | 0.46 mg |
| Calories from fat | 0 | Iron | 0.02 mg |
| Total fat | 0 g | Potassium | 10 mg |
| Carbohydrates | 3 g | Magnesium | 0.35 mg |
| Protein | 0.03 g | Vitamin A | 0.09 mcg |
| Fiber | 0.16 g | Vitamin C | 0.50 mg |

Combine the 2 cups water, sugar, and 2 ta-blespoons lemon juice in a large saucepan over medium-high heat, and cook for 3 to 4 minutes or until the mixture comes to a boil, stirring fre-quently. Using a slotted spoon, transfer the apples to the saucepan and cook for 1 to 2 minutes or until the mixture comes to a boil. Transfer the apples to a sieve placed over a bowl; drain well.

Place the apples on a baking sheet lined with parchment paper or a silicone baking mat. Pat the apple rings dry with a double layer of paper towels. Bake for 1 hour or until the apple rings are dry. If the apple rings are not dry after an hour, turn off the oven and allow them to dry in the oven. The apple rings can be stored in an airtight container for up to 3 days.

# Berries on a Skewer

*A beautiful yet easy-to-prepare garnish that adds a rich color to most smoothies.*

### 2 SKEWERS

½ cup raspberries, blueberries, cranberries, or
   blackberries

2 (6-inch) wooden skewers

Thread five to six berries of your choice on each skewer.

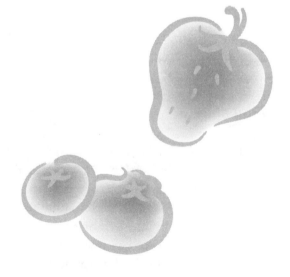

| | | | |
|---|---|---|---|
| Calories | 15 | Calcium | 7 mg |
| Calories from fat | 2 | Iron | 0.18 mg |
| Total fat | 0.17 g | Potassium | 47 mg |
| Carbohydrates | 4 g | Beta Carotene | 12 mcg |
| Protein | 0.28 g | Vitamin C | 8 mg |
| Fiber | 2 g | Folic Acid | 8 mcg |

# Candied Orange Rinds

*These are colorful and sweet garnishes that nicely complement most smoothies in both taste and appearance. This recipe is somewhat time-consuming, but the orange rinds can be prepared days in advance. For a more elegant (and indul-gent) effect, the Candied Orange Rinds can be dipped in melted chocolate\* or made into spirals\*\*.*

### 24 RINDS

2 navel oranges

4 cups cold water

2 teaspoons coarse salt

2 cups granulated sugar

1 cup cold water

Using a fork, prick the oranges all over. Cut the oranges into quarters and peel away the flesh. Remove as much of the white part as possible.

Combine the 4 cups water and salt in a large bowl, and add the orange rinds. Push down on the orange rinds with a spoon to completely submerge them in the water. Cover the

| | | | |
|---|---|---|---|
| Calories | 10 | Calcium | 3 mg |
| Calories from fat | 0.04 | Iron | 0.02 mg |
| Total fat | 0.00 g | Potassium | 4 mg |
| Carbohydrates | 3 g | Beta Carotene | 5 mcg |
| Protein | 0.03 g | Vitamin A | 0.84 mcg |
| Fiber | 0.21 g | Vitamin C | 3 mg |

surface of the water with a piece of plastic wrap; set aside for several hours or overnight.

Combine the sugar and 1 cup water in a large saucepan over moderately high heat; stir the mixture with a wire whisk until it comes to a boil and the sugar dissolves. Drain the orange rinds, and add them to the saucepan, turning them in the mixture until they are coated. Reduce the heat to low, and simmer the orange rinds for 45 minutes. Remove the saucepan from the heat, allowing it to sit at room temperature for 2 hours or until the syrup cools. When cool, pour the syrup and orange rinds into a large bowl. Cover the surface of the syrup with a piece of plastic wrap, and leave at room temperature for several hours or overnight.

Remove the orange rinds from the syrup with a slotted spoon, and place them on a cake rack set over a sheet of waxed paper to catch any drippings. Allow the orange rinds to sit for 24 hours, then slice each one on the diagonal into ¼-inch thick strips. The candied orange rinds can be stored in an air-tight container for up to 2 weeks.

**\*To make Chocolate-Dipped Candied Orange Rinds,** melt 2 to 3 ounces semisweet chocolate. After rinds are cut and dried, dip half to three-fourths of each rind in the chocolate, shake off the excess chocolate, and place them on a piece of parchment paper for 15 minutes, or until set.

**\*\*To make Candied Orange Spirals,** instead of cutting the orange into quarters, remove the peel from the orange in one whole strip (don't be discouraged if it breaks), starting at the top and working your way around until you get to the other end, making a free-form spiral. Using scissors, trim the orange rind and cut into strips ⅛- to ¼-inch wide.

# Caramelized Sugar Shards

*These versatile garnishes add a whimsical touch to most smoothies. They can be shaped into almost any design you desire and are stunningly easy to make. You can also dip each shard in melted chocolate for an even more dramatic presentation.*

12 TO 16 SHARDS

½ cup granulated sugar

2 tablespoons cold water

Line a baking sheet with parchment paper, and lightly coat it with a nonstick vegetable spray.

Combine the water and sugar in a medium heavy saucepan; bring to a boil over medium heat. Continue to cook for 6 to 7 minutes or until mixture turns golden in color, occasionally swirling the pan. Remove the saucepan from the heat and allow it to sit for 2 to 3 minutes.

Slowly pour the caramel mixture in a free-form pattern onto the baking sheet and allow it to cool. When cool, break the caramelized mixture into irregular triangular shapes. The shards can be stored in an airtight container for up to 3 days.

| | | | |
|---|---|---|---|
| Calories | 32 | Fiber | 0 g |
| Calories from fat | 0 | Calcium | 0.08 mg |
| Total fat | 0 g | Iron | 0.00 mg |
| Carbohydrates | 8 g | Potassium | 0.17 mg |
| Protein | 0 g | | |

# Chocolate Bags

*Once you make these Chocolate Bags, you will want to make them again and again. They are delicious filled with a decadent smoothie, mousse, ice cream, or fresh fruit. These bags can be made weeks in advance and stored in an airtight container in the freezer until ready to serve.*

## 2 BAGS

2 small paper bags*

6 ounces semisweet chocolate, melted

Trim the bags with a pair of scissors so they measure 3 inches tall. Open the bags to form a rectangle. Divide the chocolate between them, and, working quickly, use a spoon or pastry brush to brush the chocolate up from the bottom to completely coat the sides and corners, putting extra chocolate in the corners to make them firm. Smooth the chocolate on the bottom and make sure there are no bare spots. Place the bags on a plate and freeze for at least 1 hour.

Remove one bag at a time from the freezer, and, working from the bottom, carefully unfold the paper and pull it away from the chocolate. Place the unfilled Chocolate Bags on an attrac-

| | | | |
|---|---|---|---|
| Calories | 407 | Calcium | 27 mg |
| Calories from fat | 230 | Iron | 3 mg |
| Total fat | 26 g | Potassium | 310 mg |
| Carbohydrates | 54 g | Magnesium | 98 mg |
| Protein | 4 g | Vitamin D | 77 IU |
| Fiber | 5 g | Folic Acid | 3 mcg |

tive dessert dish in the refrigerator (or freezer) until ready to use.

*Most supermarkets have specialty coffee sections where fresh coffee beans can be purchased by the pound. Special bags that come in a variety of sizes are provided for purchasing these coffee beans. Or try shopping at a store such as The Container Store, which offers a variety of small bags for gifts. I prefer a bag with a base that measures 2½ to 3½ inches.

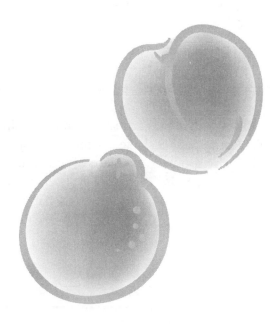

# Chocolate-Covered Spoons

*These whimsical spoons add a festive touch to a dessert or a rich flavor to a cup of coffee. They also make a lovely gift when individually wrapped in cellophane.*

### 4 SPOONS

*1 ounce semisweet chocolate, broken into four pieces*

*4 plastic, silver, or stainless steel demitasse spoons or teaspoons*

*4 feet gold cord for bow (optional)*

Place the chocolate in a cup and cook in the microwave on high for 1 to 2 minutes, stirring every 30 seconds. Dip each spoon in the melted chocolate and gently shake to remove any excess. Place the spoons on a piece of waxed paper to harden. When the chocolate has set, tie the gold cord into a bow around each handle, if desired.

| | | | |
|---|---|---|---|
| Calories | 34 | Calcium | 2 mg |
| Calories from fat | 19 | Iron | 0.22 mg |
| Total fat | 2 g | Potassium | 26 mg |
| Carbohydrates | 4 g | Magnesium | 8 mg |
| Protein | 0.30 g | Vitamin D | 6 IU |
| Fiber | 0.42 g | Folic Acid | 0.21 mcg |

# *Chocolate Curls*

*Chocolate Curls are an elegant way to elevate a smoothie to black-tie status. Once you discover how easy and fun it is to make them, you will want to decorate cakes, pies, or most other desserts with these luscious curls of rich chocolate. In fact, whenever I make Chocolate Curls, I always prepare double the amount so I can store them in an airtight container in the freezer for future use.*

1 CUP CURLS

*1 cup chocolate chips*

Melt the chocolate chips in a small heavy saucepan, covered, over low heat, stirring occasionally. (The chocolate can also be placed in a small dish, covered with plastic wrap, and set on the hot plate of a coffeemaker. Turn the coffeemaker on and the chocolate will slowly melt. Stir occasionally. Or, place the chocolate chips in a cup and cook in the microwave on high for 1 to 2 minutes, stirring every 30 seconds.)

Pour the chocolate onto a baking sheet and spread it into a 4-inch square. Smooth the top with a spatula. Allow the chocolate to sit at room temperature for 1 hour or more until it is relatively firm. With a cheese slicer that has a flat

| | | | |
|---|---|---|---|
| Calories | 136 | Calcium | 9 mg |
| Calories from fat | 77 | Iron | 0.89 mg |
| Total fat | 9 g | Potassium | 103 mg |
| Carbohydrates | 18 g | Magnesium | 33 mg |
| Protein | 1 g | Vitamin D | 26 IU |
| Fiber | 2 g | Folic Acid | 0.85 mcg |

blade and a slot at the bottom, press the blade flat on the chocolate and slide it across to make curls. If the chocolate is too soft, allow it to sit for 10 to 15 minutes, testing it every now and then. You will know when it is the right consistency, because this method creates beautiful curls.

Humidity and temperature are major factors in the timing. Do not make these in a humid or hot environment. Additionally, any broken chocolate may be melted again and reset. Store the Chocolate Curls in an airtight container in the refrigerator or freezer.

# Chocolate-Dipped Marshmallows

*Chocolate-Dipped Marshmallows transform an ordinary dessert into a spectacular one. They can be used on cupcakes, ice cream sundaes, and smoothies.*

### 4 MARSHMALLOWS

2 ounces semisweet or milk chocolate, broken into 8 pieces

4 marshmallows

4 (6-inch) skewers

Melt the chocolate in a small saucepan, covered, over low heat until melted, stirring until smooth. (The chocolate can also be placed in a small dish, covered with plastic wrap, and set on the hot plate of a coffeemaker. Turn the coffee maker on and the chocolate will slowly melt. Stir occasionally. Or, place the chocolate in a cup and cook in the microwave on high for 1 to 2 minutes, stirring every 30 seconds.) Place a marshmallow on a skewer so it is firmly in place with the point sticking almost through the top. Holding on to the free end of the skewer, dip

| | | | |
|---|---|---|---|
| Calories | 57 | Calcium | 2 mg |
| Calories from fat | 19 | Iron | 0.24 mg |
| Total fat | 2 g | Potassium | 26 mg |
| Carbohydrates | 10 g | Magnesium | 8 mg |
| Protein | 0.43 g | Vitamin D | 6 IU |
| Fiber | 0.43 g | Folic Acid | 0.28 mcg |

the top half of the marshmallow into the choco-late, allowing the excess to drip back into the pan while gently twisting the skewer with the marshmallow in the upside down position. Next, turn the skewer so the marshmallow is pointing up, and place the free end of the skewer into a glass so the marshmallow can dry without touching anything. Repeat with remaining marshmallows. Store the marshmallows in an airtight container.

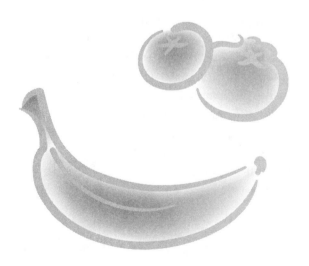

# Chocolate-Dipped Tortilla Triangles

*These triangles are so delicious, you might want to make extra. With or without the chocolate, the triangles are fabulous as a garnish, an accompaniment to coffee, or a snack.*

## 12 TRIANGLES

2 tablespoons unsalted butter, melted

1 tablespoon brown sugar

¼ teaspoon cinnamon

1 (8-inch) flour tortilla

2 ounces semisweet chocolate, broken into eight pieces

Melt the butter in a small saucepan over medium-low heat. Add the brown sugar and cinnamon, and blend well. Brush the mixture on one side of the tortilla. Place the tortilla on a parchment-lined baking sheet. Cut the tortilla into 8 triangles, and bake in an oven preheated to 350 degrees F for 10 minutes or until crisp. Cool until the chocolate is set.

| | | | |
|---|---|---|---|
| Calories | 46 | Calcium | 4 mg |
| Calories from fat | 26 | Iron | 0.25 mg |
| Total fat | 3 g | Potassium | 19 mg |
| Carbohydrates | 5 g | Magnesium | 4 mg |
| Protein | 0.48 g | Vitamin A | 18 mcg |
| Fiber | 0.30 g | Folic Acid | 5 mcg |

Melt the chocolate in a small saucepan, covered, over low heat until melted. (The chocolate can also be placed in a small dish, covered with plastic wrap, and set on the hot plate of a coffee-maker. Turn the coffeemaker on and the chocolate will slowly melt. Stir occasionally. Or, place the chocolate in a small bowl and cook in the microwave on high for 1 to 2 minutes, stirring every 30 seconds.)

Dip the *wide* ends of the tortilla triangles, ½-inch up, and place each one on a piece of waxed or parchment paper to set. Store the triangles in an airtight container.

# *Chocolate Hearts*

*Once you have mastered the technique for making Chocolate Hearts, you might try making butterflies, dragonflies, or fancy triangles. The trick is to make sure that the chocolate lines meet. To make a butterfly, for example, form the body first, then attach wings by piping three intersecting loops on each side of the body.*

### 2 HEARTS

*2 ounces semisweet chocolate, broken into eight pieces*

Melt the chocolate in a small saucepan, covered, over low heat until melted. (The chocolate can also be placed in a small dish, covered with plastic wrap, and set on the hot plate of a coffeemaker. Turn the coffeemaker on and the chocolate will slowly melt. Stir occasionally. Or, place the chocolate in a cup and cook in the microwave on high for 1 to 2 minutes, stirring every 30 seconds.) Allow the chocolate to cool for a few minutes so it just begins to thicken.

Spoon the chocolate into a parchment cone or disposable pastry bag with a ⅛-inch opening cut at the tip. Create a 3-inch heart on a piece of

| Calories | 102 | Calcium | 7 mg |
|---|---|---|---|
| Calories from fat | 57 | Iron | 0.67 mg |
| Total fat | 6 g | Potassium | 78 mg |
| Carbohydrates | 13 g | Magnesium | 24 mg |
| Protein | 0.89 g | Vitamin D | 19 IU |
| Fiber | 1 g | Folic Acid | 0.64 mcg |

parchment paper. Fill in the heart with squiggly lines, or make straight lines up and down and across each other. Place the hearts in the freezer for 1 hour. Remove the hearts from the parchment paper and use them as garnishes as directed. The hearts can be kept in the freezer in an airtight container for up to 3 months.

# Chocolate Shavings

*For those special occasions when an indulgence is in order, imagine a black-tie smoothie topped with a dollop of whipped cream covered with Chocolate Shavings. It takes no time at all to create the shavings, and they can be prepared days in advance and then stored in an airtight container in the refrigerator or freezer.*

2 TABLESPOONS SHAVINGS

*Semisweet, milk chocolate, or white chocolate*

The easiest way to make chocolate shavings is to use large chunks of chocolate broken off of candy bars that are sold by the pound. Candy stores or gourmet shops usually have chunks of chocolate that are already broken, wrapped, and ready for purchase. However, if the chunks are unavailable, all supermarkets sell 8-ounce boxes of semisweet or white chocolate that are packaged in individual 1-ounce squares.

Hold the chocolate in your left hand, and use a swivel vegetable peeler in your right hand to move the peeler toward yourself, pressing it against the side of the chocolate. Continue this process until you have the amount of chocolate

| | | | |
|---|---|---|---|
| Calories | 136 | Calcium | 9 mg |
| Calories from fat | 77 | Iron | 0.89 mg |
| Total fat | 9 g | Potassium | 103 mg |
| Carbohydrates | 18 g | Magnesium | 33 mg |
| Protein | 1 g | Vitamin D | 26 IU |
| Fiber | 2 g | Folic Acid | 0.85 mcg |

shavings you need. Depending on the chocolate, some of the shavings may look like tiny curls, some may be larger, while others may not have any curls. Store the chocolate shavings in an air-tight container.

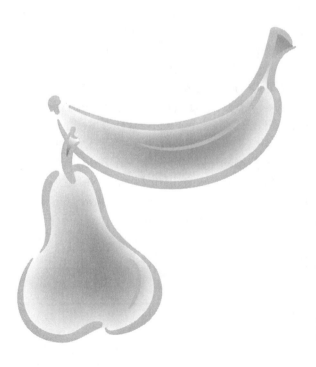

# Cinnamon-Coated Fusilli

*This garnish provides a delightful way to add a whimsical touch to a special smoothie, ice cream sundae, or almost any dessert.*

### 8 FUSILLI

*8 gourmet fusilli pasta*

*Oil for frying*

*2 tablespoons plus ½ teaspoon\* cinnamon-sugar*

Line a baking sheet with a double layer of paper towels. Set aside.

If the pasta is *U*-shaped, break each one into two equal pieces. Each piece should be about 9 inches in length. Pour enough oil in a medium fry pan to come 1 inch up the side of the pan. Place the pan over medium-high heat for at least 2 minutes or until the oil registers 350 degrees F. Place four pieces of pasta in the oil, and fry for 1 to 2 minutes or just until they begin to brown. (The fusilli will continue to brown after they are removed from the oil.) Using tongs, transfer the fusilli to the prepared pan and immediately

| Calories | 27 | Calcium | 1 mg |
| Calories from fat | 11 | Iron | 0.13 mg |
| Total fat | 1 g | Potassium | 5 mg |
| Carbohydrates | 4 g | Magnesium | 1 mg |
| Protein | 0.39 g | Vitamin E | 0.36 IU |
| Fiber | 0.09 g | Folic Acid | 7 mcg |

sprinkle with cinnamon-sugar. Allow the fusilli to cool. Store the Cinnamon-Coated Fusilli in an airtight container.

*To make cinnamon-sugar, thoroughly combine 2 tablespoons granulated sugar with ½ teaspoon cinnamon.

# Cinnamon Wonton Crisps

*These crispy, intensely flavored wontons are certain to become one of your favorite ways to garnish a smoothie or any other creation you can conjure up just to have an excuse to make them. They are so good!*

### 4 CRISPS

1 cup corn oil

4 wonton skins

Cinnamon-sugar, to taste*

Heat the corn oil in a small, heavy saucepan over moderately high heat until the oil registers 350 degrees F.

Fry one wonton skin at a time, turning it over with tongs after 6 to 7 seconds on each side or until golden brown. (The wonton crisps will continue to brown after they are removed from the oil.) Using tongs, transfer the wonton crisps to a pan lined with paper towels, and immediately sprinkle with cinnamon-sugar. Allow the Cinnamon Wonton Crisps to cool. Store them in an air-tight container for up to 2 days.

| | | | | |
|---|---|---|---|---|
| Calories | 62 | Calcium | 5 mg |
| Calories from fat | 32 | Iron | 0.30 mg |
| Total fat | 4 g | Potassium | 7 mg |
| Carbohydrates | 7 g | Magnesium | 2 mg |
| Protein | 0.79 g | Vitamin A | 0.34 mcg |
| Fiber | 0.19 g | Folic Acid | 7 mcg |

*To make cinnamon-sugar, thoroughly combine 2 tablespoons granulated sugar with ½ teaspoon cinnamon.

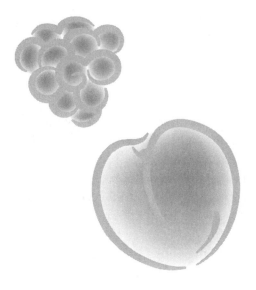

# Crisp Banana Wafers

*These crispy wafers are simply made of pureed ba-
nanas that are baked in a slow oven until the
mixture becomes brown and crisp. When cool, they
are broken into irregular pieces that can be used to
adorn any of the smoothies found in this book. The
wafers are a delicious adornment that can also be
used with other desserts, such as a dish of ice cream,
mousse, or sorbet.*

### 12 TO 16 WAFERS

*2 medium bananas, cut into 1-inch pieces*

Preheat the oven to 200 degrees F.

    Place the bananas in the work bowl of a
food processor fitted with a metal blade (or a
blender), and process for 45 seconds or until the
bananas are pureed. Spoon the pureed bananas
in the center of a baking sheet lined with a sili
cone baking mat. Using a metal spatula, spread
the puree evenly into a rectangular shape, about
1/16-inch thick. The layer should almost cover the
mat. Bake the banana puree for 2½ to 3 hours or
until brown and completely dry. Remove the

| | | | |
|---|---|---|---|
| Calories | 18 | Calcium | 1 mg |
| Calories from fat | 0.85 | Iron | 0.06 mg |
| Total fat | 0.09 g | Potassium | 70 mg |
| Carbohydrates | 5 g | Beta Carotene | 9 mcg |
| Protein | 0.20 g | Magnesium | 6 mg |
| Fiber | 0.47 g | Folic Acid | 4 mcg |

pan from the oven, place another baking sheet over the baked banana, and invert the pan. Gently remove the silicone pad and allow the baked banana to cool for 30 minutes to an hour. When cool, break the baked banana into irregular triangular shapes. The Crisp Banana Wafers can be stored in an airtight container for up to 3 days.

# Espresso Brittle Shards

*These richly coffee-flavored shards are very similar in taste and texture to peanut brittle.*

### 12 SHARDS

1 tablespoon espresso beans (or instant espresso coffee)

½ cup granulated sugar

2 tablespoons cold water

1 tablespoon butter

Line a baking sheet with a piece of parchment paper. Set aside.

If using espresso beans, place them in a food processor fitted with a metal blade or in a coffee grinder, and process until the beans are finely chopped. (The beans can also be left in the coffee bag and crushed with a mallet or rolling pin.)

Combine the sugar and water in a small heavy saucepan over high heat. Allow the mixture to boil for 4 to 5 minutes or until it turns light amber in color, swirling the pot occasion-

| | | | |
|---|---|---|---|
| Calories | 42 | Calcium | 1 mg |
| Calories from fat | 9 | Iron | 0.03 mg |
| Total fat | 0.96 g | Potassium | 21 mg |
| Carbohydrates | 9 g | Magnesium | 2 mg |
| Protein | 0.08 g | Vitamin A | 9 mcg |
| Fiber | 0 g | Vitamin D | 0.66 IU |

ally (do not stir). Using a wooden spoon, blend in the crushed coffee beans and cook for 1 minute. Remove the saucepan from the heat and whisk in the butter. Pour the mixture onto the prepared baking sheet. Tilt the sheet to make a 9- to 10-inch circle of the mixture. It does not have to be perfectly round. When the brittle has cooled, break it into large, triangular pieces. Store the brittle in an airtight container.

# Fruit Skewers

*Fruit Skewers make an attractive garnish when they are inserted into a smoothie or balanced across the rim of a glass or when the smoothie is served in a glass on a plate and the skewer is placed beside it. Moreover, the fruit is a delicious complement to the smoothie. The combination of fruits is infinite, so please use any of your favorites.*

2 SKEWERS

2 grapes

2 stemless maraschino cherries

2 pineapple wedges

2 melon balls*

2 strawberries

2 (6-inch) wooden skewers

Alternate threading the fruit on the skewers, ending with the strawberry sitting on the point. The Fruit Skewers can be kept refrigerated in an airtight container for up to 2 hours.

*You will need a melon ball scoop to make the melon balls. It has two differently size rounded spoons on each end and is available in gourmet food shops or

| Calories | 37 | Calcium | 8 mg |
|----------|-----|----------|------|
| Calories from fat | 3 | Iron | 0.27 mg |
| Total fat | 0.36 g | Potassium | 135 mg |
| Carbohydrates | 9 g | Beta Carotene | 282 mcg |
| Protein | 0.47 g | Vitamin A | 47 mcg |
| Fiber | 1 g | Vitamin C | 20 mg |

the kitchen section of grocery or hardware stores. However, you can also cut cubes of melon, and the garnish will remain just as attractive.

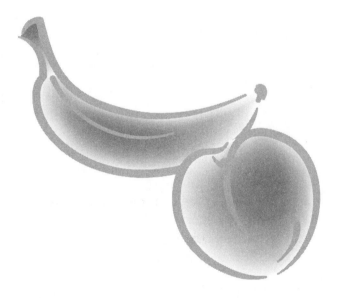

# Lemon and Cranberry Twist

*This versatile garnish can be made with an orange and blueberry, lemon and blueberry, lime and cranberry, and on and on—any combination that interests you.*

### 2 Twists

2 lemon slices (or orange), each cut ¼-inch thick and halved

4 cranberries (or blueberries)

2 (6-inch) wooden skewers

Thread a cranberry on a skewer, almost to the middle of the skewer. Place a lemon half on a plate so it looks like a *C;* push the skewer through the skin near the cut end, pass it *over* the flesh to the other side of the lemon, and push it through the skin. Thread another cranberry on the skewer, placing it close enough to the lemon half so it slightly curls between the two cranberries. Repeat with the remaining lemon half, but place it on the plate so it looks like a backward *C.* When the skewer is completed, the lemon halves should form an *S* shape.

| | | | |
|---|---|---|---|
| Calories | 4 | Calcium | 2 mg |
| Calories from fat | 0.24 | Iron | 0.05 mg |
| Total fat | 0.03 g | Potassium | 12 mg |
| Carbohydrates | 1 g | Beta Carotene | 2 mcg |
| Protein | 0.09 g | Vitamin C | 4 mg |
| Fiber | 0.32 g | Folic Acid | 0.79 mcg |

# Lemon, Lime, and Cherry Boat

*This simple garnish adds a colorful twist and sparkle to a basic smoothie. It can be placed directly on the surface of the smoothie or balanced across the edge of the glass.*

### 2 BOATS

*2 slices of lemon, cut ¼-inch thick*

*2 slices of lime, cut ¼-inch thick*

*2 maraschino cherries with stems*

*2 toothpicks*

It is best to use a lemon and lime that are equal in size. Otherwise, cut several slices from each fruit until there are two slices of equal size for each boat.

Place a lemon slice on a dish, followed by a lime slice, and topped with a cherry in the center. Hold the fruit in one hand so it forms a *C* shape, and thread a toothpick through one side of the lemon rind, then the lime, then the cherry, and, lastly, the other side of the fruit slices, making sure the garnish is neatly secured.

| | | | |
|---|---|---|---|
| Calories | 14 | Calcium | 4 mg |
| Calories from fat | 0.30 | Iron | 0.08 mg |
| Total fat | 0.03 g | Potassium | 16 mg |
| Carbohydrates | 4 g | Beta Carotene | 2 mcg |
| Protein | 0.12 g | Vitamin C | 5 mg |
| Fiber | 0.36 g | Folic Acid | 1 mcg |

# Lemon, Lime, and Orange Wheels

If you are fortunate enough to have a garnishing set that includes a food decorator tool or canalling knife, follow the given instructions. If these tools are unavailable, then you will find that this technique, taught to me by my mother, is quite simple and requires only a fork.

## 8 WHEELS

*1 lemon, lime, or orange*

Using a fork, start at one end of the fruit, and move the fork down to the other end, slightly piercing the skin. This will make a pierced line in a complete circle. Turn fruit slightly and repeat this process around the entire fruit. Remove the ends and cut the fruit into ¼-inch thick slices. To hang the wheel over the rim of a glass, make a slit by cutting through the peel and halfway into the flesh. Fit the slit over the rim of the glass.

| | | | |
|---|---|---|---|
| Calories | 2 | Calcium | 2 mg |
| Calories from fat | 0.19 | Iron | 0.04 mg |
| Total fat | 0.02 g | Potassium | 10 mg |
| Carbohydrates | 0.67 g | Beta Carotene | 1 mcg |
| Protein | 0.08 g | Vitamin C | 4 mg |
| Fiber | 0.20 g | Folic Acid | 0.77 mcg |

# Marbleized Chocolate Shards

*When white and dark chocolates are drizzled to-gether, they become a spectacular marbleized creation that can add an artistic dimension to your favorite smoothie.*

## 12 SHARDS

*4 ounces white chocolate, coarsely chopped*

*2 ounces semisweet chocolate, coarsely chopped*

Line a baking sheet with parchment paper.

Melt the white chocolate in one small heavy saucepan and the semisweet chocolate in another heavy saucepan, covered, over low heat, stirring occasionally. (The chocolates can also be placed in separate small dishes, covered with plastic wrap, and set on the hot plate of a coffeemaker. Turn the coffeemaker on and the chocolates will slowly melt. Stir occasionally. Or, place the chocolates in separate cups and cook in the microwave on high for 1 to 2 minutes, stirring every 30 seconds.)

Using a large spoon, drizzle the melted semisweet chocolate in a free-form lattice or

| | | | | |
|---|---|---|---|---|
| Calories | 74 | Calcium | 20 mg |
| Calories from fat | 40 | Iron | 0.17 mg |
| Total fat | 4 g | Potassium | 44 mg |
| Carbohydrates | 9 g | Magnesium | 7 mg |
| Protein | 0.75 g | Vitamin D | 4 IU |
| Fiber | 0.28 g | Folic Acid | 2 mcg |

zigzag design to cover a 10-inch square. Allow the chocolate to set for 1 minute. With a clean spoon, quickly drizzle the melted white chocolate over the semisweet chocolate. Gently spread the white chocolate with a metal spatula until it evenly covers the semisweet chocolate. Allow the chocolate to cool and harden completely for at least 1 hour.

Lift the chocolate with a small spatula and break off free-form triangles, or shards. Store the Marbleized Chocolate Shards in an air-tight container in the refrigerator or freezer for several days.

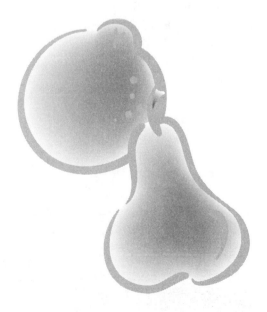

# Melon Balls on a Skewer

*You will need a melon ball scoop to make the melon balls. It has two different-sized rounded spoons on each end and is available in gourmet food shops or the kitchen section of grocery or hardware stores. However, you can also cut cubes of melon, and the garnish will remain just as attractive.*

## 2 SKEWERS

½ cantaloupe, honeydew, or watermelon, seeded

2 (6-inch) wooden skewers

Using the melon ball scoop, scoop out balls. Thread about three to five balls on each skewer. The Melon Balls on a Skewer can be kept refrigerated in an airtight container for up to 2 hours.

| | | | |
|---|---|---|---|
| Calories | 14 | Calcium | 5 mg |
| Calories from fat | 1 | Iron | 0.09 mg |
| Total fat | 0.12 g | Potassium | 128 mg |
| Carbohydrates | 3 g | Beta Carotene | 795 mcg |
| Protein | 0.36 g | Vitamin A | 133 mcg |
| Fiber | 0.33 g | Vitamin C | 17 mg |

# Orange, Lemon, and Cherry Combo

*This combo looks spectacular when it is placed on the rim of a glass.*

### 2 COMBOS

2 orange slices, cut ¼-inch thick

2 lemon slices, cut ¼-inch thick

2 maraschino cherries with stems

4 mint leaves (optional)

Make a slit in the fruit by cutting through the peel and halfway into the flesh of the orange and lemon slice. If using mint, place two mint leaves in each hole of the cherry where the pit was removed (if the pit remains, cut a small slit in the top). Cut a slit on the opposite side of the cherry. Fit the slit of the orange slice over the rim of a glass, then place a lemon slice beside the orange, and finally place the cherry beside the lemon.

| | | | |
|---|---|---|---|
| Calories | 20 | Calcium | 8 mg |
| Calories from fat | 0.37 | Iron | 0.06 mg |
| Total fat | 0.04 g | Potassium | 40 mg |
| Carbohydrates | 6 g | Beta Carotene | 8 mcg |
| Protein | 0.23 g | Vitamin C | 13 mg |
| Fiber | 0.59 g | Folic Acid | 6 mcg |

# Pineapple, Banana, and Cherry Charmer

*Like many garnishes, this one can be made with a variety of ingredients. For example, the cherry can be replaced with a carrot slice, the parsley can be traded for a carrot top sprig, and a small round of kiwi can be used instead of the banana.*

### 2 CHARMERS

1 tablespoon lemon juice

2 pineapple wedges, with skin and cut $\frac{1}{4}$-inch thick

2 banana slices, with skin and cut $\frac{1}{4}$-inch thick

2 small parsley sprigs

2 stemless maraschino cherries

2 (6-inch) wooden skewers

Lightly brush the pineapple and banana with lemon juice to prevent them from turning brown.

Thread a wedge of pineapple on a skewer, about $\frac{1}{3}$ up the skewer. Place a banana slice beside the pineapple, followed by the stem of a parsley sprig wrapped around the skewer, and finally by the cherry. Repeat with the remaining skewer.

| | | | |
|---|---|---|---|
| Calories | 31 | Calcium | 5 mg |
| Calories from fat | 2 | Iron | 0.20 mg |
| Total fat | 0.26 g | Potassium | 87 mg |
| Carbohydrates | 8 g | Beta Carotene | 15 mcg |
| Protein | 0.31 g | Magnesium | 8 mg |
| Fiber | 0.78 g | Vitamin C | 11 mg |

# Pineapple Chips

*This garnish can elevate pineapple smoothies, and many others, to a new dimension. The chips are deliciously sweet and look sensational when inserted into a smoothie. This is also a perfect garnish for a dish of sorbet, ice cream, or mousse.*

## ¼ Cup Chips

1 fresh pineapple, top, bottom, sides, and core removed

1 cup granulated sugar

1 cup cold water

Using a mandoline or vegetable slicer, if possible, thinly slice the pineapple into horizontal rings, about ⅟₁₆-inch thick. With patience, the pineapple rings can be sliced with a knife. Place the pineapple rings in a shallow roasting pan. Set aside.

Combine the sugar and water together in a small, heavy saucepan over moderate heat, and bring to a boil, stirring occasionally. Pour the hot mixture over the pineapple rings, and cover the pan with aluminum foil.

Place the pan over two stove burners; cook over low heat for 15 minutes. Remove the pan

| | | | | |
|---|---|---|---|---|
| Calories | 23 | Calcium | 2 mg |
| Calories from fat | 1 | Iron | 0.10 mg |
| Total fat | 0.11 g | Potassium | 29 mg |
| Carbohydrates | 6 g | Beta Carotene | 3 mcg |
| Protein | 0.10 g | Magnesium | 4 mg |
| Fiber | 0.31 g | Vitamin C | 4 mg |

from the burners, allowing the pineapple rings to cool to room temperature.

Once the pineapple rings are cool, place them on a baking sheet lined with a silicone sheet, and bake in an oven preheated to 225 degrees F for 60 to 90 minutes or until they turn golden brown.\* Allow the pineapple chips to cool before storing them in an airtight container for up to 2 days. The Pineapple Chips will become crisp as they cool.

\*As soon as the Pineapple Chips are baked, they can be kept whole, formed into a rolled tuile shape, or cut into wedges.

\*The Pineapple Chips can also be made by thinly slicing the pineapple into rings and placing them on a double thickness of paper towels. Pat the tops of each pineapple ring with paper towels, and then transfer them to a baking sheet lined with a silicone mat. Sprinkle ¼ teaspoon granulated sugar over each ring, and bake in an oven preheated to 350 degrees F for 60 to 90 minutes or until golden brown. Continue as directed.

# Pineapple, Orange, and Cherry Blossoms

*The impressive attractiveness of this garnish belies its simplicity. It is also a delicious taste treat after the smoothie is gone.*

### 2 BLOSSOMS

4 pineapple leaves, about 2½ inches long

2 wedges of pineapple, each with skin and cut ¼-inch thick

2 slices orange, each with skin and cut ¼-inch thick

2 stemless maraschino cherries

2 (6-inch) wooden skewers

Thread a cherry on a skewer, almost to the middle. Thread an orange behind the cherry, followed by a pineapple wedge, and finally by the two pineapple leaves. Repeat with the remaining skewer.

| | | | |
|---|---|---|---|
| Calories | 38 | Calcium | 10 mg |
| Calories from fat | 2 | Iron | 0.17 mg |
| Total fat | 0.20 g | Potassium | 77 mg |
| Carbohydrates | 10 g | Beta Carotene | 11 mcg |
| Protein | 0.32 g | Vitamin C | 15 mg |
| Fiber | 0.90 g | Folic Acid | 9 mcg |

# Pineapple Spears

*Pineapple Spears perched on the rim of a glass add a tasty, tropical flair to a smoothie.*

### 4 SPEARS

I small pineapple

Cut the pineapple in half, lengthwise. Cut one half of the pineapple into quarters, and make an incision parallel with the core. Place the Pineapple Spear on the rim of the glass. (The remaining pineapple can be cut into cubes and placed in the freezer to be made into a smoothie.)

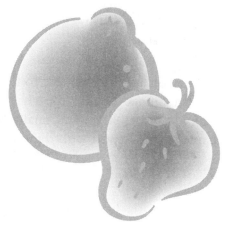

| | | | |
|---|---|---|---|
| Calories | 29 | Calcium | 4 mg |
| Calories from fat | 2 | Iron | 0.22 mg |
| Total fat | 0.25 g | Potassium | 67 mg |
| Carbohydrates | 7 g | Beta Carotene | 7 mcg |
| Protein | 0.23 g | Magnesium | 8 mg |
| Fiber | 0.71 g | Vitamin C | 9 mg |

# *Pirouettes*

*Serving a smoothie garnished with a Pirouette cookie is the ultimate way to deliciously adorn these delectable treats. Although there are a host of delightful commercially made pirouettes that come in assorted sizes and flavors, I prefer to make my own. This versatile recipe is very easy to prepare, and once you perfect the process, I hope you will be encouraged to experiment with other ways to shape the dough.* \*

12 PIROUETTES

4 tablespoons unsalted butter, at room
   temperature

2 tablespoons clover honey

½ cup powdered sugar

½ cup flour

1 egg white, beaten until foamy

Preheat oven to 375 degrees F.

Place the butter and honey in a medium bowl, and beat with a handheld electric mixer on medium speed for 1 minute or until well combined. Add the powdered sugar and flour, and beat on low speed for 2 to 3 minutes or

| | | | |
|---|---|---|---|
| Calories | 84 | Calcium | 2 mg |
| Calories from fat | 35 | Iron | 0.27 mg |
| Total fat | 4 g | Potassium | 13 mg |
| Carbohydrates | 12 g | Vitamin A | 36 mcg |
| Protein | 0.88 g | Vitamin D | 3 IU |
| Fiber | 0.15 g | Folic Acid | 8 mcg |

until smooth and creamy. Add the egg white, and beat just until incorporated.

Spoon 1 rounded tablespoon of the batter on each half of a nonstick baking sheet or a pan lined with parchment paper or a silicone mat. Spread the batter with the back of a spoon into a 5-inch circle. (Do not worry if the batter looks uneven—it will even out during the baking process.) Bake for 6 to 7 minutes or until the edges begin to turn golden brown. Allow the cookies to cool for 1 minute, then lift each with a metal spatula to loosen and quickly roll up each cookie into a tight cylinder or cigar shape. Place the cookies, seam side down, on a cake rack to cool completely. Repeat the process with the remaining batter. The cookies can be stored in an airtight container for up to 3 to 5 days or frozen for a couple of weeks.

**\*To make cones:** Spoon a scant tablespoon of batter into two 3-inch circles on the baking sheet and bake for 5 to 6 minutes or until the edges are golden brown. After 1 minute, remove the cookie with a metal spatula and shape it into a cone, making sure to leave a large enough opening at the top for the ice cream. (To make larger cones, use rounded table-spoons of batter to make 5- to 6-inch circles.) Repeat six times until you have a total of twelve cones.

**\*To make cookie cups:** Spoon rounded tablespoons of batter into two 5- to 6-inch circles on the baking sheet, and bake for 6 to 7 minutes or until the edges are golden brown. After 1 minute, remove the cookies with a metal spatula, and immediately drape them over a large glass or custard cup, gently pleating the sides to make a cup shape. Allow the cookies to cool before removing them from the glass or cup. Repeat six times until you have a total of twelve cookies.

# Strawberry Fans

*Strawberry Fans add a nice touch of color when placed on the rim of a glass, as well as being a tasty treat.*

## 2 FANS

*2 whole firm strawberries, unhulled*

Using a very sharp knife, make vertical cuts through the strawberry, starting from just below the top and cutting through to the bottom. Make about five to six very thin cuts, depending on the size of the strawberry. Place the strawberry on a plate and carefully spread the slices apart to resemble an opened fan. Slip a Strawberry Fan over the rim of each glass.

| | | | | |
|---|---|---|---|---|
| Calories | 4 | Calcium | 2 mg |
| Calories from fat | 0.40 | Iron | 0.05 mg |
| Total fat | 0.04 g | Potassium | 20 mg |
| Carbohydrates | 0.84 g | Beta Carotene | 2 mcg |
| Protein | 0.07 g | Vitamin C | 7 mg |
| Fiber | 0.28 g | Folic Acid | 2 mcg |

# White Chocolate–Dipped Strawberries

*These strawberries are a delicious way to dress up any smoothie. They also look fabulous placed on the top rim of a cake or served with your favorite ice cream, mousse, or other dessert.*

## 8 STRAWBERRIES

1½ ounces white chocolate, coarsely chopped

½ teaspoon vegetable shortening

8 strawberries, unhulled

Place the white chocolate in a small saucepan, covered, over very low heat. Cook until the chocolate has melted, stirring occasionally. (The chocolate can also be placed in a small dish, covered with plastic wrap, and set on the hot plate of a coffeemaker. Turn the coffeemaker on, and the chocolate will slowly melt. Stir occasionally. Or, place the chocolate in a small bowl and cook in the microwave on high for 1 to 2 minutes, stirring every 30 seconds.) Remove the choco-

| | | | |
|---|---|---|---|
| Calories | 41 | Calcium | 15 mg |
| Calories from fat | 19 | Iron | 0.13 mg |
| Total fat | 2 g | Potassium | 68 mg |
| Carbohydrates | 5 g | Beta Carotene | 5 mcg |
| Protein | 0.51 g | Vitamin C | 18 mg |
| Fiber | 0.74 g | Folic Acid | 7 mcg |

late from the heat, and whisk in the vegetable shortening until smooth.

Dip the pointed end of each strawberry into the chocolate, halfway up, allowing the excess to drip back into the pan. Place the dipped strawberries on a cookie sheet lined with waxed paper, and refrigerate for 5 minutes to set the chocolate. The strawberries can be kept at room temperature for up to 4 hours.

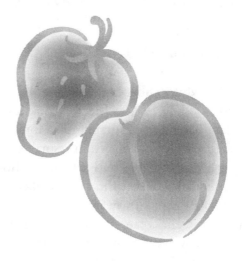

# Index

# International Conversion Chart

These are not exact equivalents: they have been slightly rounded to make measuring easier.

## Liquid Measurements

| American | Imperial | Metric | Australian |
| --- | --- | --- | --- |
| 2 tablespoons (1 oz.) | 1 fl. oz. | 30 ml | 1 tablespoon |
| ¼ cup (2 oz.) | 2 fl. oz. | 60 ml | 2 tablespoons |
| ⅓ cup (3 oz.) | 3 fl. oz. | 80 ml | ¼ cup |
| ½ cup (4 oz.) | 4 fl. oz. | 125 ml | ⅓ cup |
| ⅔ cup (5 oz.) | 5 fl. oz. | 165 ml | ½ cup |
| ¾ cup (6 oz.) | 6 fl. oz. | 185 ml | ⅔ cup |
| 1 cup (8 oz.) | 8 fl. oz. | 250 ml | ¾ cup |

## Spoon Measurements

| American | Metric |
| --- | --- |
| ¼ teaspoon | 1 ml |
| ½ teaspoon | 2 ml |
| 1 teaspoon | 5 ml |
| 1 tablespoon | 15 ml |

## Weights

| US/UK | Metric |
| --- | --- |
| 1 oz. | 30 grams (g) |
| 2 oz. | 60 g |
| 4 oz. (¼ lb) | 125 g |
| 5 oz. (⅓ lb) | 155 g |
| 6 oz. | 185 g |
| 7 oz. | 220 g |
| 8 oz. (½ lb) | 250 g |
| 10 oz. | 315 g |
| 12 oz. (¾ lb) | 375 g |
| 14 oz. | 440 g |
| 16 oz. (1 lb) | 500 g |
| 2 lbs | 1 kg |

## Oven Temperatures

| Farenheit | Centigrade | Gas |
| --- | --- | --- |
| 250 | 120 | ½ |
| 300 | 150 | 2 |
| 325 | 160 | 3 |
| 350 | 180 | 4 |
| 375 | 190 | 5 |
| 400 | 200 | 6 |
| 450 | 230 | 8 |

# Juicing Recipes to Tingle the Taste Buds

Cold, delicious juice drinks never go out of style. They're perfect in any kind of weather and at any time of day. Most important, they're as nutritious as they are mouthwatering. *Ultimate Juicing* overflows with 125 great-tasting fruit and vegetable drinks that use the sweet, zesty juices of everything from apples to tomatoes. Inside, you'll discover a wealth of fun and easy-to-prepare recipes for the most delectable fruit and vegetable drinks imaginable, including:

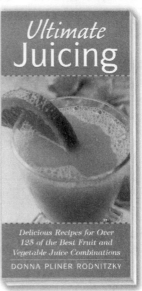

*Ultimate* **Juicing**

*Delicious Recipes for Over 125 of the Best Fruit and Vegetable Juice Combinations*
DONNA PLINER RODNITZKY

ISBN 0-7615-2576-9
Paperback / 240 pages
U.S. $12.95 / Can. $19.95

- Adam's Apple
- Berry the Hatchet
- The Beet Goes On
- Grin and Carrot
- Cool Hand Cuke
- Heard It Through the Grapefruit
- And many more!